Autism and Asperger Syndrome in Childhood

I have been working in the field of autism for decades, in capacities ranging from practitioner to researcher to trainer to lecturer.

My work has involved helping local authorities to develop services and good practice, coordinating and developing services and training for the National Autistic Society (NAS) and being part of a research team at Nottingham University. I have also spoken at a number of national and international conferences on a variety of autism-related topics.

Presently I am a senior lecturer on autism at Sheffield Hallam University. I am the course leader for the postgraduate certificate in autism and Asperger syndrome, run in collaboration with the NAS, and supervise several students at doctoral level, many of whom are autistic. I am very proud that several of my autistic (ex) students have completed their doctorates successfully. I also continue to be involved in research in a wide range of autism-related areas.

In 2011, I was awarded the Inspirational Teacher Award, in 2012 the Inspirational Research Supervisor Award and, in 2018, my third Inspirational Award. In recognition, my university presented me with the Sheffield Hallam Vice-Chancellor Award. In 2015, I was a finalist for the prestigious NAS's Lifetime Achievement Award for a Professional. In 2016, I was the winner of the NAS's Autism Professionals Award for Achievement by an Individual Educational Professional. In 2016, I was nominated and reached the finals for the Autism Hero Awards in two categories – Lifetime Achievement and Individual Professional – and won both categories.

Occasionally, I have made media appearances, including on the BBC and Radio 4, and featured in articles that have been published in the *Guardian*, the *Independent* and *The Times*. In the award-winning *Aukids* magazine, in its list of the top ten all-time favourite autism blogs, mine reached the number two spot.

In other writing, I co-wrote the ASPECT consultancy report – the largest consultation that had ever been undertaken with adults with Asperger syndrome up until that time – I have co-edited five books on autism and Asperger syndrome, I wrote *Autism and Asperger Syndrome in Adulthood* and have written various other pieces published in journals and books.

To my beautiful and patient wife, Kate: you first helped me become a happy person; you then made me an even happier person; and now you keep me happy. Don't ever stop, you lovely, lovely human. I owe you so much.

To Guy: sometimes being shoddy ain't so bad! You know I've got a bad back. You're a part of my life I could never imagine being without; thank you for being you.

To Fionn: my absolute (snow) man. A pair of 'D's you might be, but you mean the absolute world to me.

To all three: without you, I am nothing. I love you. xxx xxx xxx

Overcoming Common Problems

Autism and Asperger Syndrome in Childhood

For parents and carers
of the newly diagnosed

DR LUKE BEARDON

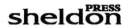

First published in Great Britain in 2019 by Sheldon Press
An imprint of John Murray Press
An Hachette UK company

1

Copyright © Dr Luke Beardon 2019

The right of Dr Luke Beardon to be identified as the Author of the Work
has been asserted by him in accordance with the Copyright, Designs and
Patents Act 1988.

A CIP catalogue record for this title is available from the British Library

Paperback ISBN 978-1-847-09492-6
eBook ISBN 978-1-847-09493-3

Printed and bound in Great Britain by Clays Ltd, Elcograf S.p.A.

John Murray Press policy is to use papers that are natural, renewable and
recyclable products and made from wood grown in sustainable forests.
The logging and manufacturing processes are expected to conform to the
environmental regulations of the country of origin.

Sheldon Press
Carmelite House
50 Victoria Embankment
London EC4Y 0DZ

www.sheldonpress.co.uk

Contents

Foreword

This is the book I've been waiting for; it will now be on the top of our recommended reading list (at Axia ASD Limited) – it is absolutely essential. I have had the pleasure and privilege of knowing and working with Luke for over 20 years now and am delighted he has now found the time and energy to write this much needed addition to the world of autism. The book clearly meets its aims regarding 'overcoming common problems' and is aimed at parents and carers of the newly diagnosed.

However, I believe it would be suitable for a much wider audience, as it clearly lays out common misunderstandings and myths that still sadly dominate many professional opinions and society as a whole. Instead it comes from a position of celebrating autism, acknowledging the enormous strength autistic individuals bring to society, without whom it would be a much less interesting place.

The book may be too much for some of the predominant neurotype to fully understand; however, as Luke himself says, 'if you cannot understand, you just need to accept [the Autistic reality]'. Another of Luke's very helpful statements is outlined in the book: 'Autism + environment = outcome'. This should be the mantra to ensure autistic individuals are not damaged or indeed destroyed, as they currently are, particularly when they have spent years and years masking in order to try to look like the predominant neurotype. The ultimate outcome for any of us is to be happy and Luke stresses this in the book, giving real-life examples as to how to achieve this.

There is an endorsement of what I call the 'Partnership Model' in contrast to the predominant 'Expert Model' seen in services. This Expert Model is also embodied in the diagnostic criteria which Luke critiques, along with a balanced look at self-identification. Autistic people need to be seen as the experts on themselves and must be listened to and enabled to have what Luke has termed 'a strong sense of self'. This book should be essential reading on any training course: for example, clinical psychology, mental health nursing, teaching and so on, and it is particularly helpful for anyone thinking about embarking on seeking, or having recently received, a diagnosis for themselves or their child. It will also be essential reading for those who would like to understand the positives and strengths of being autistic and, I hope, the future of autism.

Dr Linda Buchan, Consultant Clinical Psychologist,
Founder and Director, Axia ASD Ltd

Acknowledgements

To all those amazing autistic folk and families who have shared, and continue to share, their lives with me. You have taught me all I know.

Introduction – and welcome to autism!

So, as the chapter heading states, welcome to autism! And a very warm welcome it is, too. Whether you are reading this as someone who thinks your child may be autistic or has recently found out that he or she is, or as a sibling, grandparent or any other family member, or a keen professional looking to expand your knowledge – whoever you are, I am delighted to have you join this fabulous, intriguing, beguiling, frustrating, fascinating, wonderful, exciting, remarkable and awe-inspiring world of autism. And, yes, it can be all of those things – and far more besides! Irrespective of what you might have been told, what your current thinking is or what preconceptions anyone might have, I promise you, the list of adjectives that can describe what you will go through in the forthcoming years is pretty much endless.

Before I go any further: the title of this book refers to 'autism and Asperger syndrome[1] in childhood' – just for absolute clarification, I do not believe that autism is 'in' anything, but this book is aimed at parents of children, hence the reference to childhood. Second, autism is around to stay, it's for life, not just for childhood – just thought I'd best make that clear! Third, while the title does refer to childhood, my hope is that the book might be useful way beyond the readership of parents, so if you don't 'fit' into the category 'parent of an autistic child', don't stop reading!

A quick note on terminology

So, when I write 'I', I mean me. But while I refer to myself, what I am really doing is leaning incredibly heavily on experiences that have been so kindly shared with me over the decades – real-life

---

[1] Asperger syndrome is included in the title as many people will have this as a diagnosis and may continue to, depending on the next edition of *International Statistical Classification of Diseases and Related Health Problems* (ICD). However, as the *Diagnostic and Statistical Manual of Mental Disorders* (DSM) no longer recognizes Asperger syndrome as a diagnosis, I refer to autism from here on throughout the book

experiences of autistic children and adults, parents of autistic children and, of course, sometimes the experiences of autistic parents of autistic children.

When I write 'you', I mean you, the reader. I am hopeful that this book may be useful to a whole range of people, including professionals, but, in the main, I am imagining that my audience is the parent – so that is who I am addressing as 'you' unless I state otherwise.

When I write 'we', I am referring to society as a whole, as a collective, without singling out any specific part of that population.

When I refer to 'your child', I may switch between genders – this is for narrative flow more than anything else. I am of the opinion that there are as many autistic girls as boys, so will use 'him' or 'her' and 'he' or 'she' interchangeably. By the way, I am fully aware that the number of girls identified as autistic is way lower than is the case for their male counterparts, but this is not because girls are less likely to be autistic, but because they are just less likely to be identified as such! Also – while we're clarifying things – although I use 'child' in most cases throughout, autistic children do grow into autistic adults; many of the issues written about in the book are equally applicable to adults.

The predominant neurotype (abbreviated to PNT) is my preferred term for referring to the non-autistic population. Many people use the term 'neurotypical', but I am wary of the possible connotations of 'typical' with its potential associations with 'normal'. Autistic children are not abnormal. In fact, most autistic children are delightfully 'autistically normal', usually until others get hold of them and try to make them behave more like the PNT!

I use 'autistic child' (or sometimes 'autie') rather than 'child with autism'. This stems from the overwhelming autistic voice that asks us to do so; it also aligns with my beliefs around language and the importance of the autistic self. Autism is not an 'add-on' to the person! This particular point is explored in many written works, not least blogs written by autistic authors. My understanding is that being autistic is *intrinsic* to the person; thus, I prefer to avoid 'with autism', which, to me, suggests that autism is not an integral part of the human being.

Very importantly, when I refer to the autistic child I am doing exactly that – in other words, I am not referring to a child who has additional intellectual impairments. Any child – autistic or not – may have intellectual disabilities (or learning disabilities); autistic children will demonstrate a full range of intellectual abilities that will play a significant part in how the child experiences life. This book has its focus on children who are autistic, not children who are autistic with additional learning disabilities.[2] However, I do also know of people who have had a diagnosis of learning disability in childhood who end up demonstrating that they have no intellectual disability whatsoever – in fact, they may turn out to demonstrate high levels of intellectual ability. Being autistic can massively increase levels of anxiety, which, in turn, can lead to a child 'presenting' as less intellectually able than he or she actually is. Over time, if those anxieties decrease, it can become apparent that the original supposition of a learning disability was an error. This raises a hugely important point, about not judging a child merely based on how he or she presents. More on this later.

Last – and possibly most importantly – just because being autistic puts your child into a minority group, it by no means lessens his or her importance or place in this world. Your child need not be defined by being autistic, and you do not need to be defined by being the parent of an autistic child. It is sad, in many ways, that there is commonly a 'majority rules' kind of attitude within society: almost invariably, within a group, the autistic child will be identified as exactly that – the 'autistic one' – but not in this book! In this book, the narrative is all about the autistic population; it is the PNT that is in the minority, at least in terms of the subject matter. I certainly use 'autistic' frequently throughout the book, but I also simply refer to 'children' or 'child' – the assumption being, within this context, that those referred to are autistic. So, if I need to refer to a PNT child, then I will proactively do so. In the meantime, feel free to assume that any child I refer to will be an autistic girl or boy.

---

2 Having noted that, I believe many aspects of this book would also be invaluable to the population of individuals with the dual diagnosis of autism and learning disabilities, so I am not in any way excluding that population.

Autism and intelligence

Incidentally, intelligence has nothing to do with autism. One can be autistic and incredibly intelligent, and one can be autistic with a profound learning disability – and one can be autistic and sit anywhere in between those two states. Actually, I am not sure why I started the paragraph with 'incidentally' – it is not incidental at all, it is an important point; so many people assume that being autistic means either one has some kind of amazing savant-type skill (which, while some may, is not actually particularly common) or one has intellectual disability. These are the sorts of assumptions that are based on ignorance and should be widely ignored. Being autistic does not tell you anything about an individual's intellectual ability whatsoever.

My position on things

Clearly, what I write is my opinion and, as such, is open to challenge. However, I aim to be as 'true' as I can to all those extraordinary people who have taught me so much over the years and allowed me to formulate my own voice and opinion, in the hope that I do justice to the amazing autistic population I have been so fortunate to engage with. So my caveat, I guess, is that, while I won't constantly keep writing 'in my opinion . . .' as it would become cumbersome, do bear in mind that everything is, indeed, just that! You will soon discover that, within the autism world, there are such varying opinions – some diametrically opposed to one another – that finding any consensus is nigh on impossible. Having noted that, many people are very firm in their own beliefs – and I think that my own beliefs are absolutely justified!

. I won't go into all the reasons why you should trust me and won't bore you with my CV. Rather, read on and simply decide for yourself whether or not what I'm writing makes sense and is helpful to you and your child. Far too much is written about autism as a tragedy, a mystifying 'condition' that takes away the 'normal' child, leaving the parent bereft and mourning what could have been. Why? I don't read stories of parents of PNT children suddenly bemoaning the fact that their child isn't showing any of those gorgeous characteristics so often associated with autism. I don't hear parents saying, 'Oh, my poor child, she isn't autistic – and poor me, I'm missing out on that incredibly rich experience of parenting an autistic child' and so on. Just because parenting an autistic child brings its own challenges (which it certainly does), that doesn't mean the child herself is any 'less' or should be seen in a different light simply because she happens to belong to a minority group. Many of the challenges, as you will discover for yourself, I am sure, stem from the outside world rather than from the child herself; the problems often arise from society and its ignorance about autism – not from the autistic individual herself.

My 'position', therefore, is that autism is *not* a tragedy. Yes, autism brings its own set of problems, issues, challenges, but many of those are situated outside of the child. Being autistic need not be a problem; being autistic in a society that doesn't understand, however, that most certainly *can* be a problem.

Why read on?

So, let's get something straight from the outset: much (maybe even most) of what you might read, listen to, hear about in relation to autism is negative. This can range from the way it is represented in the media to articles in academic journals and everything in between. There is a small but growing number of voices (literally and figuratively) that counter this negative perception, and this book situates itself firmly in among them. Your child is not a disordered, impaired, diseased, dysfunctional person, despite what you may have already been told or what you may already have read. The common, current parlance for autistic children is to use the term 'autistic spectrum disorder', which is how autism is referred to in the two main diagnostic manuals. However, I do not subscribe in the least to the notion or concept that autism is a disorder – indeed, I suspect that we are doing our autistic children a huge disservice by 'branding' them in this manner.

The way in which this book is written means that you can read the chapters in any order you wish. There are very few references to other literature and it is intended to be easy to read but still well informed. Throughout the book I have included 'the autistic voice'; sometimes these are 'real' voices – stories or thoughts from autistic people I know who have given me permission to include them – and sometimes they are fictitious but based on a combination of real situations. The inclusion of 'the autistic voice' is essential as one of the crucial successes in supporting autistic children is to understand life 'through the autism lens' – that is, from the autistic perspective. In doing so, one's world can become illuminated beyond the rather narrow perspective of the majority and shine a light on the extraordinarily rich and diverse population that is autistic. Most of these sections are rhetorical questions from a parent, but with 'real' answers from the autistic child. Of course, each 'answer' is likely only to be applicable to that specific child, but the accumulation of responses throughout the book may offer you some insight into the differing perspectives of what parents and professionals 'see' and what autistic children perceive. Here is an example.

> *Parent*: I wonder why you always stare so hard at the light bulb in the porch. Why do you have to spend so much time there before coming fully into the house? It's such a pain, having to wait around for you, but when I encourage you to get a move on you seem to get so angry and lash out!
>
> *Child*: Transitions are so difficult for me. I like safety, I crave it. Being safe is so important to me. Being in the car is safe; I know what to expect. Being in the house is safe; I know what to expect. But getting to the house from the car? Mummy, it's a nightmare. The world outside always looks so different each day, it's unpredictable, the smells change all the time – it's like walking into the unknown each and every time, I hate it! But that porch light . . . hmm . . . the light's texture (yes, I can 'feel' it), the perfection of it being 'just right' – Mummy, it makes my heart melt to look at it, it takes away the strain of transition, it eases my soul. Please don't take it away from me! One day I expect I will need less time to gaze upon its wonder, but in the meantime, come share it with me, don't rush through, sit with me quietly while I suspend time and stress to ease myself from one setting to another. I love that light, Mummy, why don't you?

What this book is not

There are limitations to any book on autism – this is OK, so long as it is understood from the outset what to expect (and what not to). I could have included detailed chapters on all sorts of things, but I could also have expanded each of the chapters that I have written – in fact, each chapter could easily be a book in its own right! I fully accept that I will have left out tons of stuff that you will need as a parent; my rationale is that one aim for the book is 'setting the scene', as it were, to give a baseline upon which you can continue to build your understanding of autism as you read and find things out elsewhere.

My absolute drive for this book, though, is to support the notion of the happy autistic child. The book raises issues, concepts and notions that are sometimes taken for granted, sometimes not considered and often applied inappropriately to autistic children. The book highlights these deliberately in order to encourage a deeper reflection – to ask questions such as, 'Is this appropriate *for my autistic child?*' – and, by doing so, aims to influence practice to make it more autism-friendly and, thus, increase the chance of happy autistic kids.

A conversation from the future

I would love that, one day, this book becomes defunct. I would love it if there wasn't so much nonsense written about autism, so many beliefs that are inaccurate and demeaning to the autistic population. I would love it if our knowledge of autism was so excellent, a book such as this would reside on a shelf gathering dust. Until then, however, we have a long way to go. The following passage, ending the Introduction, is a fictitious conversation, taking place in the future.

Girl: Hello, Mummy.
Mother: Hello, darling.
Girl: Mummy, I want to ask you some questions.
Mother: OK, fire away!
[Pause]
Girl: Fire away?

Mother: Sorry, darling, silly Mummy. I meant please do ask your questions.

Girl: Oh. So why did you say 'fire away', then?

Mother: It's my fault, I sometimes forget that we have different ways of talking – it's my mistake, sorry.

Girl: That's OK, Mummy. Anyway, we were doing autistry at school – you know, the module on autism history, all about people like me but in the past – and I really didn't understand it. You're middle-to-almost old, so I thought you'd be a good person to ask. Is that OK?

Mother: [Chuckles] 'Middle-to-almost old', very funny!

[Pause]

Mother: Sorry again. Yes, of course, I will try to answer any questions you have.

Girl: OK. Well, first off, we were told that to be autistic, the children had to go and see a doctor – is that true?

Mother: Yes, dear, that's true.

Girl: But why?

Mother: So they could be told they were autistic.

Girl: But why a doctor? Don't we go to the doctor when we're ill?

Mother: Well, yes.

Girl: So why did children have to go to a doctor when they weren't poorly?

Mother: Um. Well, I guess it's because they had a very different view of autism then.

Girl: Oh. Right. Really? That's really, honestly true then – they used to think it was like being ill? I thought I'd heard wrong when we were told that they had to go to a doctor.

Mother: I'm not quite sure if it was quite like that, but, yes, children did have to go and see a doctor.

Girl: Wow. Didn't that make the kids feel bad?

Mother: I think it probably did sometimes, yes.

Girl: Well, that's stupid then. Why make kids feel bad just for being autistic?

Mother: I don't really know. I think, actually, lots of people did think it was bad to be autistic then.

Girl: How can you be bad just for being a person? That's just silly!

Mother: Yes, I agree. It does seem silly!

Girl: OK. Well, my next question is about adults. Were there really and honestly and truly adults who didn't know they were autistic until much later in life?

Mother: Yes, absolutely – really. Quite a lot of adults, actually.

Girl: How come?

Mother: Um . . . er . . . well, I suppose people didn't realize.

Girl: Well, obviously, but how can people not realize? Was it less obvious then than it is now or something?

Mother: Um, no, I don't think so. I think it's because the doctors years ago maybe didn't understand autism in the way we do today. Or some did but some didn't. Did you know that lots of them had hardly any training in understanding autism?

Girl: What? So they didn't take autistry modules like I'm doing now?

Mother: Well, no. No one did.

Girl: No one?

Mother: No, my love, those sorts of modules didn't exist then.

Girl: So how did anyone ever understand anyone else who might be a bit different?

Mother: I'm not particularly sure that understanding was seen as very important back then.

Girl: That's ridiculous – how can children be happy if they are not understood?

Mother: Well, I agree . . . but . . . I don't know how to answer that. It seems obvious now, but it didn't seem so obvious then – not to everyone, anyway. There were some people who did lots of campaigning to try and get more people to understand what it means to be autistic, but lots of people weren't especially interested.

Girl: How come?

Mother: I really don't know, darling. I really don't. Things were very different back then.

Girl: Right. OK. So, another question. Is it really true that lots of autistic children couldn't go to the same schools as other kids – and that autistic adults weren't allowed to go to work?

Mother: Well, it's definitely true that lots of autistic children didn't go to the same schools as other kids. It isn't the case that adults weren't allowed to work – more the case that they found it difficult to *access* work.

Girl: [*Frowns*] Why? That doesn't seem very fair on children like me. And autistic adults make brilliant employees, we know that.

Mother: Well, yes – they do today because there is so much more understanding of autism these days. Back then, when people didn't really understand, things were much tougher for autistic people.

Girl: So it all comes back to this understanding business?

Mother: Yes, I'd say so.

Girl: So, tell me again: why didn't people want to understand? When it seems that a better understanding would mean happier autistic people, more autistic children going to schools and adults being employed? And all it takes is what we do now – autistry modules taught by autistic teachers to all kids from day one at school, plus all the 'share my life' lessons that we all do that make school so much fun.

Mother: I don't really know. It seems so simple when you put it like that.

Girl: Mummy?

Mother: Yes, my darling?

Girl: People used to be really weird, I reckon.

Mother: Yes, now that I think about it, I have to agree.

1

Frequently asked questions

What is autism?

OK, so to start with something easy . . . or complicated, depending on which way you want to look at it! In a sense, the simplest explanation of autism is that it is a *different cognitive and sensory state* – in other words, a hard-wired difference in the way your child thinks and responds to the sensory environment. So that's it! However, the complexities lie in the individuality of the impact this has on your child – not just as a person today, but throughout life. Autism will have an impact on any one given individual in a unique manner at that particular time, and this impact is massively influenced by the environment.

The golden equation

My so-called (self-professed) 'golden equation' is:

autism + environment = outcome

What this means is that being autistic, in and of itself, cannot really tell us anything about the immediate, short-, medium- or long-term effects on the person. What can tell us something about the lived experience – the 'outcome' component in the equation – is that it is the *combination* of the person and the environment that will subsequently lead to the reality for the person. Take the following two scenarios as an example.

> First day at preschool. Well, I say 'day', but it was more like half an hour. I'd never been there before, so had no idea what to expect. The lady had come to our house and shown me some pictures, explaining to me that this was what the place looked like.

She lied.

The rooms looked totally different, with people in them and different pictures on the wall, and one room was even painted a different colour. This made me stressed the second I walked in. Then the lady asked me how I was feeling. I couldn't answer, I was too stressed and, anyway, I was such a mix of emotions that there was no way I could have answered. Some other kids – some of whom smelled really badly of wee – were there and the lady made us sit all together, even though I wanted to be as far away from them as possible. She then sang loud songs and made us clap. It hurt my ears and my hands, and the smell of the other children made me feel sick. In the end, I ran out and hid in this lovely cosy room where mops and buckets lived. I couldn't filter individual words when the lady was shouting at me through the door, so I just stayed there until Daddy came to pick me up. We were told I wasn't welcome back until I could learn to fit in. I don't know what I've done wrong.

First day at preschool. What an amazing place. The lady had come to our house and live-streamed a video of the place I was going to the next day, carefully explaining that it might look and sound slightly different by then. She told me that if I had any problems at all, then she was the one I could go to, which really reassured me. When I got there, she was waiting for me. She didn't speak much, just showed me to the room and assured me that I could sit where I liked throughout the day and didn't have to do anything I didn't want to and that I could use my headphones (ear defenders) when I liked. The other kids sat together, but I was in the corner away from their smells so didn't mind at all. When they sat and clapped, I put my 'ears' on and it made me feel all peaceful. I even plucked up the courage to gently place my hands together and the lady smiled at me and told me I was amazing and that it was great joining in. I had a brilliant time, I felt all safe and understood and can't wait to go back tomorrow.

What this demonstrates is the power of the environment. The child is the same child, irrespective of the physical environment, the support and the people within it, but the latter components clearly, in this case, made a huge difference to the child's lived experience. This is why I am fixated on the 'golden equation'!

The golden concept

Just while I'm on the subject, how about a 'golden concept' to tack on to the 'golden equation'? If anyone (parent, teacher, professional and so on) is supporting the child (in any way) and the way in which this is being done is rooted firmly in the way that 'works for everyone else' (in other words, the PNT population), then there is a high risk of it being a method that is less applicable to the autistic child. All of those 'concepts' that are based on preconceptions around PNT kids will not apply in the same way to your child who – of course – is not PNT. Perhaps one common example is:

Teacher: Look at me when I'm talking to you!

This is based on the fact that most of the PNT believe that 'looking' equates to 'attention', so an indication that the child is attentive might be the fact that he is looking at the speaker. If a child is not appearing to be attentive, then a good 'strategy' is to ask for the child to look. There are even schools where staff praise 'good looking'. This is absolutely understandable so long as the strategy remains within the PNT. If applied to the autistic child, however, the risk of it becoming problematic will increase. This is not to suggest that it won't work for any autistic children (though I do suspect that it is unlikely to 'work' for very many in the same way that it does for the PNT, if any at all), but it certainly can cause problems that the PNT may not be aware of. Here are some (internal) responses from a few autistic children to that very 'command'.

- 'OK, I'll look at you, sure. Only now that I'm looking at you I literally cannot hear a word you're saying so don't have a go at me when I don't follow your instructions. I can either look or listen, I can't do both at the same time.'
- 'Why should I look at you? You've got me perplexed now. In fact, you've confused me so much with this inane command to look at you when you're talking to me that my brain has switched off

from what you're saying to contemplate why on earth you've said it in the first place. The very last thing I will do is look at you!'

- 'So I look when you're talking, then what? I look away? Where do I look then? I'm concentrating so hard on working out when you're talking to me so I can look that I can't possibly follow what you're actually saying, but at least I'm doing as I'm told.'

As you can see, the command here will not have the required (or expected) outcome. In my view this is an example of how the PNT might assume that 'the same rules apply', but the reality may be very different for the autistic child. So be (very) wary of anyone who is suggesting that the way in which you engage with your child (in any way) is based on PNT assumptions about 'what works and what doesn't'. Actually, and rather frustratingly, you won't always be able to rely on other parents who might be generous in their advice, stemming from what worked for them and their child. While it might be useful, it is not a guarantee that what works for one autie kid will work for all! Of course, some advice might be incredibly useful – just don't make any assumptions. One of the major issues that becomes clear in the above example(s) is that the reaction of the PNT – if they lack an insight into the child's internal responses – may simply be that they think the child is being deliberately disobedient or obtuse in some way; in other words, not only has the adult given a 'request' or command from a PNT perspective that is inapplicable to the child, he or she has then judged the reaction of the child from a PNT point of view. This is wrong on every level, but with the result that the autistic child is deemed to be 'in the wrong'.

What is autism? (continued)

Back to the question 'What is autism?' Many of the diagnostic criteria are problematic to me for three main reasons:

- some are based on behaviour;
- they are extremely negative in the way that they are constructed;
- some seem to me to be flawed in relation to my understanding of autism.

I will cover the latter later on in Chapter 3 in the sections on myths.

Basing any criterion on behaviour has to be an issue: *there is no such thing as an autistic behaviour*. In other words, there isn't anything that an autistic child might do that isn't seen in the PNT. There may be all sorts of behaviours that are more common, absolutely, but as they are not exclusive, they cannot be deemed 'autistic'. Autism is situated within the brain. Behaviour will clearly be influenced by whether one is autistic or not, but should it ever be used as a diagnostic criterion if there is no such thing exclusively as autistic behaviour? So I refute criteria that are based on behaviour. In this sense, we can certainly suggest that, currently, it is impossible definitively to identify autism! That isn't to suggest that autism does not exist (it clearly does), nor that we should not be identifying it (we clearly should), just that there is no definitive 'test' with an empirical 'answer'.

I had a go at a definition of autism for another book and came up with the following:

> Autism refers to a neurotype that leads to a cognition that is qualitatively different from that of the predominant neurotype (PNT) in the way that information specific to communication, social interpretation and interaction is processed and understood; and to a perceptual reality of the sensory environment that differs considerably from one individual to the next.

I was identifying that autism impacts the thinking style and processing of the individual, including sensory profiles, and that the key areas of cognitive differences in comparison with the PNT relate to communication, social interpretation and interaction. While I am still pleased with this definition, subsequently a rather better one has come to light, in Dr Julia Leatherland's doctoral thesis, completed at Sheffield Hallam University:

> Autistic individuals share a neurological type, which is qualitatively different from that of non-autistics, and which will necessarily impact, both positively and negatively, on aspects of their thinking and learning; sensory processing; social relational experiences; and communicative style, abilities and

preferences. An autistic person's experience of and ability to be successful in the world will be dependent on the closeness or compatibility between their individual profile of skills and requirements and their physical and social environment. Levels of sensitivity to environmental factors vary between individuals and within the same individual over time, so that the presentation of autism is ever changing. A person's neurological type, however, remains constant, and being autistic is a lifelong identity.

Both of these definitions identify autism without any negative, pejorative language, and I think that they are both valuable and useful as a basis for understanding autism.

Can autism be cured?

As noted above, in Dr Leatherland's definition, autism is a lifelong identity. There is a huge amount of debate about this: should we, as a society, even be attempting to seek a cure for what some – myself included – argue is an extremely valuable group of individuals within the general population? Yet money is still being spent on genetic identification. This sounds scarily suspicious to me. What if an autism gene was identified? What would we do about it? Why are we even looking for it? My concern is that if such a gene were to be discovered, it could be used as an option for decreasing the autistic population and, to me, that would be a tragedy beyond comprehension. My feelings aside, I also think (suspect very strongly) that it would have a massively negative impact on the world.

The actual concept that autism *should* be 'cured' is, to me, an extremely odd one. Autism is part of who a person is – and is not, as noted, in and of itself a negative. It may be *made* negative by stigmatization, ignorance, lack of understanding, erroneous assumptions, inaccurate media portrayals, bad education, poor research – the list could (and does) go on – but, again, this is not a true reflection of autism.

Back in the day, being left-handed was seen as a negative and people were 'cured' of being left-handed. In reality, they were never 'cured' – their behaviour was remodelled to reflect that of right-handed folk. Rather than continue this very strange practice, society decided simply to educate itself and recognize that, while being left-handed might in some circumstances put one at a disadvantage, in and of itself there was nothing in the slightest wrong with it. In fact, the golden equation can be applied here just as well as it can to the situation for your autistic child. Thus, if a left-handed child is put in an environment where everything is set out for right-handed kids, the child will be at a disadvantage. Change the environment – make all the facilities and equipment left- *and* right-handed-'friendly' – and, all of a sudden, the disadvantage disappears and the result is a happy left-handed child. I see no difference between seeking a 'left-handed gene' and an autism one in relation to a cure. In brief, I find the idea abhorrent and appalling.

I absolutely accept that being autistic can bring a whole array of problems, but I am firmly of the belief that the answer to those problems is not to try and make a person not autistic; the answer lies in ascertaining the true core of those problems and focusing on them. I also happen to believe that many of the obstacles for autistic children stem not from being autistic but from a combination of factors, not least co-morbid conditions. Being autistic does not preclude one from having any other co-morbidity. In fact, there are some overlaps in terms of diagnostic frequency – for example, attention deficit or deficit hyperactivity disorder (ADD/ADHD), dyslexia and dyspraxia are all common co-morbid diagnoses. If you were to identify the spectrum of neurodiversity, you would find all sorts of overlaps. What is more problematic is when there is a co-morbidity that can impact very negatively on quality of life, the issue then being that some people might assume that autism itself is the defining factor making life negative. I agree wholeheartedly that, for some, being autistic and having co-morbid diagnoses can lead to extremely poor quality of life, but I simply cannot accept that being autistic in and of itself will automatically lead to the same outcome.

I know many very happy, contented autistic people. The idea that these wonderful humans do not have a place in this world is not one that I subscribe to. Of course, there are many deeply unhappy autistic people, but I remain convinced that the cause of their unhappiness is not being autistic per se, but society not providing the appropriate support, whatever that may be.

Where does autism come from?

Right, so, following on from the above, the likelihood is that, in the main, autism is, in fact, genetically linked. This does not mean that the parent(s) are necessarily autistic themselves, but the chances of a parent of an autistic child being autistic him- or herself is higher than for a parent of a non-autistic child. Indeed, very many adults who realize they are autistic do so as a direct result of their child being identified! As this book refutes the concept of a cure and is about celebrating, understanding and supporting autistic children rather than looking backwards, I shall keep this section very brief. Suffice to say, it is extremely unlikely that there is anything you (as parents) have done to 'cause' autism, aside from providing your genetic make-up. You may not even have done anything that way – there are plenty of children for whom there appears to be no genetic link at all.

What will the future hold for my child?

I have no idea – and neither does anyone else. Do *not* believe any scaremongers. Do *not* drown yourself in negative statistics. Do *not* listen to anyone at all who professes to know what the future will hold for your child. No one has a crystal ball, no one can see into the future, so no one knows what will happen in time. For some reason, once a child is identified as autistic, people come up with all sorts of extremely unhelpful suggestions as to what this might mean. It is simply ludicrous. Being autistic, for your child, will certainly influence his or her life's experiences, but it will not dictate them. You may hear, for example, worrying statistics about autistic people not being well represented in employment as adults. Forget it. Do not apply them to your child. Those statistics are not based on your child – they are based on past generations and likely will have absolutely no relevance whatsoever to your situation. As an aside – and this is an important one – there is very little point in those statistics anyway, as they only apply to people with a diagnosis. We don't actually know the real figure, as we know for sure that loads of adults remain undiagnosed. For all we know, they may be very happily employed. Thus, we simply do not know, so be very wary of statistics!

This raises a very important point: one of comparison. For some utterly illogical and bizarre reason, people often seem drawn to comparing autistic people with one another, as if this is in some way appropriate. You will quite possibly already have experience of this. The classic response when you are telling someone about your child being autistic is so often, 'Oh, really? My neighbour's cousin's dog's friend's owner knew an autistic child once . . .', as if that bears any relevance whatsoever to your child! Your child is your child. There is no point comparing him or her to anyone else.

What is far more important than trying to predict the future is to prepare yourselves (you and your child) for it. Never 'set the bar' – who knows what the future might hold? Also, if you believe the hype and set a bar too low, it might be that your child will never aim higher. Irrespective of how your child develops during child-hood, never make any assumptions about what might happen next. Here are some examples of how things turned out for some autistic children. In these cases, I would like to point out that they are all real and nowhere near as isolated as you might think.

- **The child who 'couldn't read'** Throughout all his school years his teachers told his parents that their child was intellectually impaired and would never read. At the age of 18, he got so fed up with everyone telling him he couldn't read that he decided to teach himself. He now devours books that most people would not be able to decipher.
- **The child who 'couldn't learn'** OK, so I'm not referring to any one specific person here – there are so many of them! The number of adults I know who say that they were told, or their parents were told, 'Your child can't learn' or 'Your child can't be taught' who ended up doing degrees later in life or doctorates as an adult . . . the multi-millionaires I meet who left school at 16, told that they would never amount to anything – these indi-viduals are plentiful. It should not be assumed that just because learning does not happen in the conventional ways it means

that a child is *unable* to learn. Far more often it is the teaching style that is of little benefit to the autistic child – but changes in the teaching can have a massive positive impact on the learning!

- **The child who 'couldn't speak'** Well, not until she could! Children who are non-verbal as kids do not always remain that way. Some kids will speak perfectly well, just at a later stage than their non-autistic peers. While some may remain non-verbal, it is not always the case.

- **The child who 'couldn't socialize'** Not, that is, until he met the right person to socialize with, then he wouldn't stop socializing! Being of a different neurotype may make it harder to find the 'right' person (or people) to engage with successfully, but it doesn't mean that person doesn't exist.

The list could go on for a seriously long time. Suffice to say, avoid anyone who ever suggests that what happens today is a direct indicator of what will happen tomorrow. It simply is not true. We don't tend to do this with non-autistic children, so why do it simply because one has a diagnosis?

My point earlier about statistics is a really important one. As we currently know that there is a significant disparity between what we *expect* the numbers of autistic people in the world to be (or any given specific country, city, town, village . . .) and the *actual* numbers that have been recorded, then we simply cannot say with any conviction whatsoever what life patterns are for most autistic people (sources vary, but today it is safe to suggest that the autistic population is more than 1 per cent of people in general, yet the numbers of children and adults identified as autistic are not close to that percentage). We do know all sorts of things – such as that if we don't support autistic children in an autism-friendly way, then it could cause harm – but what we categorically do not know is where all the autistic adults are, nor what they are doing. We do know about some, but absolutely not all. If we take this, then add the fact that, anyway, generations will experience life very differently just because society changes so quickly, then the idea that one could judge a child's future based on current adult experience becomes objectively nonsensical.

Will my child succeed?

As above, I have no idea and, again, nor does anyone else. What I would suggest, though, is to be very careful about what you identify as 'success'. For an autistic child, success may look very different from success for the PNT. We are fairly poor – despite protestations – at recognizing individual needs. We tend to make all sorts of assumptions based on the majority, which is a dangerous game to play when we are referring to a minority group! After all, should the same 'rules' apply when it comes to a population who, by definition, are cognitively different from the PNT? The answer is very clearly 'no', yet autism is actually very infrequently taken into account when considering what aspects such as 'success' or 'well-being' actually mean.

There are, without a shadow of a doubt, very many happy autistic adults. It must be noted that there are also deeply unhappy autistic adults, but if the outcome can be so very different, with a common denominator being 'autism', then it stands to reason that being autistic will *not* automatically lead to being either happy or unhappy. What is absolutely critical is the addition to the autism of the environmental factors along the way – again, that 'golden equation'. So, you could expand on the same conceptual equation and hypothesize the following:

autism + lack of understanding = poor outcome
autism + good understanding = positive outcome

I believe absolutely that – as is the case with pretty much any child – the better the understanding a parent has of the child, the better he or she can support that child and the lower the risk, then, of negative outcomes in the longer term. Getting to know an autistic child means coming to understand just how autism impacts that particular child. What is of the utmost importance always is remembering that your child will share all sorts of things with other autistic kids and yet will also experience the world in ways that differ, sometimes considerably, from those of other autistic children.

So what can't my child do that the PNT child can?

Well, there is pretty much nothing that your child cannot do simply because he or she is autistic. I like thinking about a sentence that starts off, 'Being autistic means that a child can't . . .' and pondering what could follow on that is 100 per cent applicable to all autistic children. I suspect that there are a few things, but the one that springs to my mind is, 'Being autistic means that a child can't be not autistic', which sums it up nicely! There is nothing that an autistic child is unable to do. Some things may be harder (even considerably harder) and some things may well be tons easier than they are for non-autistic children. Just as is the case for all children, though, the factors that influence ability go way beyond what particular neurotype one is.

2

Identification

Identification, not diagnosis

I dislike the term 'diagnosis'. You may already have noticed that I tend to use 'identification' in lieu of 'diagnosis'. The reason for this is, I am of the firm belief that part of how we should be supporting autistic children along a happy and healthy pathway (and by 'healthy' I am very much referring to emotional and mental happiness in this context) is to de-medicalize being autistic. Currently, the whole process of identification is very much rooted in the medical model of disability, which to me is absolutely incorrect. Let's just take a peep at one of the main diagnostic manuals, the *Diagnostic and Statistical Manual of Mental Disorders*. The language within the 5th edition (DSM-5, 2013) includes words such as:

- disorder
- deficit
- impairment
- abnormal
- symptoms
- disturbances.

Charming, eh? So your child has to be disordered, have deficits, impairments, symptoms, disturbances and be – above all – abnormal. No wonder parents feel crushed when their child goes through this often brutal process and comes out the other side with these labels attached to him or her. The frustrating thing is that we don't need to use any of these extremely pejorative terms. We don't need to medicalize autism. Autism is not a medical condition, it's simply a different way of thinking about and processing the world. The trouble is that society has this erroneous sense of what it is to be 'normal' and those who do not fit neatly into this category are considered 'abnormal', which is just plain mean!

Imagine if we were to go back in time and categorize women as 'abnormal men', labelling them as such. After all, women 'lack' all sorts of 'male characteristics', but are they impaired, disordered and abnormal? The idea is so ludicrous that it barely warrants a mention and yet, in this day and age, we are still doing a similar thing to autistic children on a daily basis. Rather than simply identifying autistic children as autistic (which is extremely important), we are using diagnostic terminology that paints a very bleak (and false) picture indeed. What implications are there for the child? What does this process and use of language tell the parents about their loved one? What knock-on effects might there be of all of this on the future?

The entire process, from start to finish, could be viewed as flawed. At a subconscious level (at the very least), autism is regarded as 'wrong'. In order to get a 'diagnosis', parents usually have to see a GP in the first instance, but we tend to go to our GP to find out what is wrong with us! We go to determine how to be fixed. We go to get a cure for whatever is 'wrong' with us. Is this really the message we should be giving to parents who suspect their child might be autistic? If we perpetuate the notion that autism is essentially a second-class normality, then we are doing a huge injustice to autistic children and their families.

Using the term 'identification' is, to me, far more appropriate and, indeed, accurate. Current parlance is not even to use the term 'autism' – it's 'autistic spectrum disorder' (more on this later). Which is likely to have a less negative impact on the family: being identified as autistic or being diagnosed with autistic spectrum disorder? Ultimately, they tell the same story, but in vastly different ways.

Pros and cons of identification

Should we be identifying children as autistic? Absolutely, yes. Knowledge is key – in fact, I would go so far as to suggest that denying someone from being identified as autistic could have repercussions ranging from frustration and irritation right through to severe damage. The latter we see in adults who have not been identified and forced to live in a way not according to their genuine selves because no one has recognized that they are, in fact, autistic. Pros include:

- you knowing who your child is;
- your child knowing who he or she is;
- wider family and society knowing who your child is;
- protection from the law;
- understanding that usual rules may not apply.

Cons include:

- people not believing you;
- people subsequently making daft assumptions based simply on the identification;
- people having different expectations – again, just based on the identification, not the child;
- people not seeing beyond the identification.

You may see a pattern emerging from the 'cons' list: they are all about other people and ignorance related to autism. So, in a sense, they are not cons of an identification – they are an indication of just how little autism is understood. As a parent, it can be unbearably frustrating to hear comments or responses to the declaration of your child being autistic that are simply ridiculous. So, to prepare you for what you might encounter, here are some comments that you may hear, along with some suggested mental responses in italics (probably best to keep them to yourself, as people don't like to be told how daft their comments actually are!).

- 'Autistic, eh? So what's his special ability?' *I said autism, not superhero.*
- 'But how can she be? She's a girl!' *Yes, thank you. I had noticed that my daughter is female, and I have also noticed that she is autistic. The two are not mutually exclusive. It's not my fault that historically people thought that only boys could be autistic.*
- 'Oh, no – how awful. I'm so sorry.' *What on earth are you sorry for? What is so awful? You do realize that you are basically telling me that my gorgeous child is a tragedy – which is really not a very nice thing to hear!'*
- 'Autistic – so does he have to go to a special school?' *Why? Why,*

why, why? Why would being autistic automatically mean that you think he needs to go to a special school?

- 'So does that mean he shouldn't really be playing with my daughter?' *Really? Are you serious? He's known your daughter all his life. He hasn't suddenly morphed into a different child just because we finally managed to get an identification!*

- 'Hmm, are you sure? I know an autistic bloke from work and he's nothing like your son.' *So you're telling me some random stranger from a totally different background who is thirty years older than my five-year-old child are in no way similar. Wow, what a surprise?!*

- 'OK, so she's really good with numbers?' *No, she's not. I don't know where you got your information from, but not all autistic children are number geeks. Before you ask, she's also rubbish with computers, useless at art and has a shocking memory. Next question?*

- 'But how can he talk, then?' *Why would being autistic mean he can't talk? Are you actually serious?*

- 'I don't know, I saw that programme the other day and he doesn't seem very much like the autistic character to me.' *Yes, and I saw a programme the other day and you're nothing like the non-autistic adult male either. So what's your point again?*

- 'How can he be, he's just so lovely and cute?' *Yes, he is. I have no other response to make aside from one that would no doubt put you off me for life. Suffice to say, I will keep it in my head instead.*

- 'Er, is it catching?' *OK, I'm off now . . .*

Suffice to say, you will need to arm yourself against some of the ignorance that you will encounter along the way. Of course it's not all doom and gloom – there are plenty of people who do have a better understanding of autism than the average person, but we are still a long way off from being where we need to be.

How to get an identification and what to expect

It's nearly impossible to find a neat and easy way to get your child identified. Although some (limited numbers of) families manage to go through the process easily, swiftly and with a positive outcome, there are some families who have to wait years, have to continually ask to be re-referred and who simply do not seem to be able to get an appropriate conclusion.

The main influencing factor in getting an appropriate identification is to be prepared. Having a written record of all your thoughts about why you feel it may be necessary to 'assess' for autism – against the diagnostic criteria if at all possible (however horrible this might seem) – can be hugely beneficial. Most importantly, remember that you know your child better than a clinician who might only see him for a few hours – you've known your child all his life! It is easy to see the clinician as the 'expert', but it is rather more likely that you are the expert when it comes to knowing your own child. This doesn't mean necessarily that you have more expertise in autism, but you will have more expertise in 'your child', so don't lose sight of that along the way.

It is likely that you will have to undergo the medicalized process of 'diagnosis', so it's well worth mentally preparing for it. Part of this is making sure – as far as is possible – that you are prepared for an assessment to focus on some of the difficulties that your child might be perceived to have, which might make for a very negative experience for you (and your child) overall. Always bear in mind that we are still in a culture of pathologizing autism, so the very process of identification is rooted in a medical 'impairment'-based model. While I do not align myself with this model, it must be recognized that this is the world we live in, so steel yourself and prepare for the worst! Remind yourself that it is a necessary means to an end. Of course, you may come across a professional whose view differs from that of the majority, in which case the whole process may be rather more pleasant than is often reported.

Telling your child

First things first – should you tell your child that he's autistic? In all probability, yes. The question really should be, 'When and how?' I tend to think that there need to be three factors – three ticks against a checklist, if you like – before going ahead with 'the chat'. They are:

1 communicative ability
2 conceptual ability
3 motivation.

Communicative ability pretty much speaks for itself (excuse the pun). Your child needs to have the receptive communication skills in order to have the chat in the first place.

Conceptual ability is another thing entirely. This important point goes beyond chatting about an autism identification and should be taken into account for all communications with any autistic child. As adults, we often assume that our own concepts of language are similar enough to our child's that when we use language it is meaningful *in the same way* as we understand it. This may be the case, but it is by no means guaranteed for the autistic child, for whom language may develop somewhat differently. If this is the case, then pre-empting this and teaching abstract concepts in an autism-friendly manner is crucial long before you engage with your child about him being autistic.

I suggest that the key concepts affiliated with language terms that need to be understood in a non-negative way are those of 'difference' and 'minority'. This means that when you come to chat about being autistic and you use those terms, your child will already have an appreciation of them – and if you do manage to develop a conceptualization that being different and being in the minority does not equate to anything negative, then his first introduction to being autistic – vitally – will not be negative either.

My favourite way of developing understanding of conceptual language is simply through play. You can use whatever your child is interested in, but the concept is the same – you want to be identifying 'difference' and 'minority' without negativity at all times. Say your child likes animals, the following could be a scenario at the zoo.

You: Wow, there are a lot of elephants at this zoo, aren't there?
Him: Yes, I counted and there are a lot.
You: But we only saw one giraffe.
Him: Yes, just one.
You: Elephants are different from giraffes, aren't they?
Him: Yes, of course.
You: But do you like both giraffes and elephants, even though they are different?
Him: Yes, of course.

You: And do you like the giraffe any less, just because there was only one?

Him: Again, of course not – why would I like it any less just because there's only one?

You: Indeed!

This sounds oh so simple – and it is! Yet, you have successfully managed to develop a clear notion of 'difference' and the fact that just because something is in the minority and is different doesn't make it 'lesser' in any way. You can expand on this with questions such as, 'What are the similarities between giraffes and elephants?', 'What are the differences?', 'What are the pros and cons of being each animal?', 'Would it be difficult being a giraffe living among elephants and being expected to fit in?' and so on. The way in which such simple 'games' can develop, taking on quite complex notions and concepts, can be hugely powerful. When it comes, then, to chatting about autism, you can refer back – 'So, like that giraffe at the zoo, you are in the minority, and it might be more difficult as a result and, yes, you're different – but no less of a being than that giraffe was who was well outnumbered by elephants.' You can take this even further when it comes to things like communication and skills. Elephants have different communication and skill sets compared to giraffes, but no one skill set or form of communication is superior to another. Elephants might get on really well in an elephant-friendly environment, while the sole giraffe might struggle. Take the elephant, however, and pop him into a giraffe-friendly environment and it's a whole different story. All of these are analogous to what it's like to be autistic!

Last, motivation: your child needs to have some level of wanting to know, and this can stem from all sorts of different experiences. Sometimes it's a query that arises from finding something either much easier than peers or perhaps somewhat harder. This can lead into an explanation as to why that might be. Other factors that might influence the beginnings of a chat are noting how certain characters on TV are 'different' in some way – other family members, even the autistic character in *Sesame Street*!

One final – but important – aspect to note is that if you can include something concerning a passionate interest in a positive manner in relation to being autistic then so much the better. I am convinced that a child's first notion of being autistic is absolutely critical to his or her subsequent feelings about it. Having an introduction in a positive manner (as opposed, for example, to some types of assessments) could be influential in a positive way. So, if your child is a nature enthusiast, do your homework and identify well-known autistics involved in nature and bring that into the conversation. The same can be done for almost any area of interest, from music to film to science, however tenuous it might be. 'Using' a passionate interest in a positive manner as regards the autism 'chat' might be a powerful tool towards a positive notion of the autistic self.

Simply put: I am of the school of thought that when I hear of an autism identification, the word that springs to mind is 'congratulations', *not* 'commiserations'.

The importance of a strong sense of self

Being autistic is, by definition, being different from the majority of other kids. It is deeply disturbing to me that we as a society do not do enough to identify autistic children as soon as we could nor as effectively as we should. To understand oneself as an autistic person is a valuable and potentially life-changing notion that should never be denied a child. These diary entries articulate the point.

Dear Diary,
I hate school. I hate everything about it. I hate the noise, the smells and the sounds. I simply find it so difficult to cope with it all. I try so hard to play with the other kids, and they're not mean, but I just don't know what to do. I feel under so much pressure to do what they do, yet they all seem to know exactly how to be with each other without even trying, whereas for me I spend my entire day trying to figure it all out without getting anywhere. It's exhausting, terrifying and deeply worrying. Most of all, Diary, I hate myself. If I wasn't so useless I would be able to fit in like the others, and school wouldn't be a problem. How come they all breeze along without a care in

the world, while I wake up every morning in despair at having to face the same torments all over again?

Compare that with the following entry.

Dear Diary,
Another successful day at school for me – hurrah! Made it to the gates and went straight round the side along the quiet route to avoid the crowds, spent a lush few minutes in the little garden at the back where I could chill and gear up for the day. Another little autie chap was there as usual, and as usual he flapped at me in a friendly manner and I flapped back. I could hear the other kids playing together before school, but I'm not bothered. I might want to join in one day, but for today I'm happy being me and I understand why. Lessons were great; as always, I worked hard and enjoyed learning new things. Of course, playtime is always harder than lessons, but it's not a huge problem. I get to eat on my own so I don't have to put up with the vile canteen, so I don't go hungry; and spending time in the library is almost as good as spending time in the lessons! It's kinda cool being autistic – different, for sure, but being allowed to do things my own way, and knowing why I need to, and not feeling bad coz I'm not the same as the others – such a relief! I remember hating being me, when all the time I was thinking I had to be the same as everyone else. Now I know why I am the way I am – wow, it's such a relief.

If one is autistic and one doesn't know about it, or if one knows one is autistic but doesn't really know what that actually means, this may lead to a poor sense of self. Not only that, but the temptation is to keep comparing self to others. This is massively problematic, as if the population against which one is comparing oneself is a 'false' population – that is, one not appropriate for comparison – then the 'results' will be flawed. *There is simply little or no point in comparing the autistic self to the PNT*: doing so will only leave a bad taste in the mouth! But if a child doesn't know any better, then this is exactly what he or she will do. More about this will be covered in Chapter 6.

Who else to tell

So you have your child's identification; what do you do next? First, take some time. Don't rush into anything. You have all the time in the world; there is no mad rush to act immediately. Once you have told people, you can't 'untell' them! Disclosing can be both a welcome relief and a potential nightmare. And it almost all depends on how those you tell react. It may be useful to tell one person at a time to gauge reactions and learn from anything useful in terms of his or her reaction – it can be surprising how people react. It might even be worth preparing something like a quick 'question and answer' sheet that you can give so that others can read up sensible things about your child before either bombarding you with questions or going on to the internet and deciding they know more about your child than you do!

Blame culture

I am not suggesting that this will happen, but in some circumstances there might be an element – for example, from grandparents – of whose 'fault' it is. There is clearly no blame to be apportioned when it comes to autism; it is literally nobody's 'fault' (or to put it more positively, no one can 'claim' to have been the sole benefactor to the wonderful autistic child!). However, some people seem desperate to identify a cause or 'point the finger'. I suspect that this is an example of not accepting and rejoicing in the autistic child, more than anything else, and it should be discouraged – it does no good whatsoever.

Impact on the wider family

No one will remain unaffected by having an autistic child in the family, which is only natural. After all, everyone is affected by a new addition to the family, autistic or not! However, siblings do need a particular mention. Whether older or younger, living with an autistic sibling is highly likely to be a different experience from living with PNT siblings (the dynamics will obviously be different again if both (or more) siblings are autistic). For example, one 'rule' that applies to the PNT child may not apply in the same way to the autistic sibling, and this needs to be explained carefully to the PNT sibling so that he or she does not feel in some way hard done by.

Similarly, the wider family will have an important role to play – the more people who are in contact with your child who absolutely accept him being autistic and needing to be accepted and supported, the better. Chapter 6 discusses the happy autistic child; having a wide network of people who comfortably and absolutely accept your child for who he is and strive to understand him will go a very long way to meeting this goal.

3

Autism theory, myths and alternative perspectives

What is autism theory?

Without wishing to state the obvious, autism theory is pretty much what it states: theory that attempts to explain autism. The problem is that there isn't any one autism theory that actually 'works' – in other words, that does, in fact, explain autism. Some theories explain some components, but there is no single theory that can be applied to all autistic children – so, in a sense, one could argue that all autism theory is moot!

In this chapter I do not aim to go into theory in any great academic depth. If you want to read up on autism theory, then please start with Dr Nick Chown's superb book *Understanding and Evaluating Autism Theory* (Jessica Kingsley, 2016). In my view, it is the best book ever written on autism theory and does a far better job than I would ever be able to do.

My book is aimed at you, the 'new' parent, so my brief introduction to theory will be less academic and more designed to provide you with some thoughts as to whether or not particular theories apply to your child.

Can autism theory explain autism?

No. As noted, autism theory cannot explain all there is to understand about autism – otherwise books like this would be unnecessary, I guess. This raises all sorts of problems, as if one accepts that some autism theory might be useful at explaining some aspects of being autistic for some kids – which is a reasonable concept to accept – then how can one decide which theory applies to which child and in what way? It's a real minefield, especially as autistic kids have a habit of changing over time (as do all kids) so what might apply one day may all of a sudden not apply a few weeks later. This isn't to suggest that autism theory has no use – good autism theory can be incredibly useful to help understand the autistic experience – but the way in which one might interpret or understand autism theory can lead to a very different understanding of the child.

Autism as a spectrum

So autism is known, pretty much globally now, as being on a spectrum (or continuum). The problem with this – at least, one of the problems – is that people have very different ideas as to what this means, so when they refer to the spectrum it might mean that they are communicating at cross purposes. My main problem with it, though, is the connotation that there is some kind of spectrum of ability or behaviour or level of autism on which one can situate an autistic child relative to other autistic children. Now, I am the first to recognize that there are professionals, autistic adults, clinicians, academics and others who do firmly believe that there is a spectrum of autism that ranges from 'mild' to 'severe'. However, I also believe that there are pretty good arguments (that I subscribe to) suggesting that at a conceptual level it is, at the very least, *unhelpful* to view autism in this way. My (fairly simple) rationale for this is that I believe it is the *impact* of autism on the individual which might be considered to be severe (or not) – and the impact, as I've mentioned once or twice already (!), is *a combination of autism and the environment*, not autism as a stand-alone component. In this sense, the impact on an individual might be severely negative in one environment, yet that person might thrive in another. His or her autism remains exactly the same, so in my view, it is the circumstances around the person (including the environment) that have changed – hence my genuine belief that autism per se is not severe, mild or otherwise. Here is an example.

> I am standing in front of a huge audience to do a keynote speech about what it means to be autistic. There are hundreds of people here, but I'm perfectly calm. I do know that my non-autistic fellow speakers are lined up behind me and that they are in varying states of nerves – I know this because I

overheard them discussing it a short while ago. One of them even said she was feeling sick – why, I have no idea. It's only talking in a monologue about something you are expert at, after all. In my view I struggle to think about anything less anxiety-inducing. I mean, look at me – all I am doing is talking about myself, which is about as easy a subject as one could ever get. One of the other speakers ascribed her nerves to the number of people in the audience – again, how weird is that? What difference does the number of people in an audience make when one is making a speech? I couldn't care less if I was speaking to one person or the whole city – it literally makes no difference to me. And yet I'm the one who apparently is severely impaired in communication!

Later . . .

I've lost it altogether. The speech was fine as far as I'm concerned – I have no idea what the audience thought about it. But without me being warned about it beforehand the organizers announced that after my talk there was to be an 'unstructured break' and I would be available to 'chat' to people if they chose to approach me. What a disaster! It was totally unexpected, I had not prepared my brain for chaotic, random interactions in which I was expected to perform to a certain standard; when people approached me they often spoke at the same time or interrupted one another; I had very little idea as to what each person even wanted – one woman simply said, 'I enjoyed that very much,' and then paused, as if I was supposed to respond in some way! I mean, what? I was surrounded by people whom I had never met, with a barrage of questions that I had not had time to prepare for, I had no idea how many people wanted to ask questions nor how long I had to answer them, thus I had no perspective on the duration of each answer I should give – even if my brain wasn't so overwhelmed that it had an answer to give. I clearly needed to escape before having a full-blown meltdown, but my abrupt departure without any vocalization as to what I was doing (my brain had entered flight mode and shut down all areas of brain activity, including speech, that were not directly needed for flight-associated purposes) led to a bunch of very annoyed, disgruntled, offended people. I am absolutely inconsolable – I thought I had been asked to do a nice, simple talk but I ended up making a total fool of myself, presumably never to be invited back.

The above example is an indication of how autism within one context can range from a positive (presumably mild or not even worth a 'grade') to having very negative – possibly even 'severe' – consequences for the same person just a few moments later. So is the person 'mildly' or 'severely' autistic? This is one of the reasons that I reject the notion of a spectrum of severity.

The next reason that I proffer is one of concept. If there is some kind of grading spectrum, then could it be possible to somehow move along it? Can one 'make' a child be less (or even more) autistic? To my mind the answer is a resounding 'no', and I see it as actually a nonsensical question. It's a bit like asking, 'Can I make this dog less dog-like?' While that may sound like a ridiculous analogy, it does in fact have some merit. One could, I guess, shave a dog, paint it to look like a cat, pop it in some clothes – whatever – to make it *appear* less like a dog, but it will still, underneath it all, be just as much a dog as it was before the surface alterations. In my view, this is very similar to what some people might argue when they suggest that such and such an 'intervention' has made a child 'less autistic', the rationale proffered being that the child behaves in a different way or talks when previously non-verbal, or whatever the distinction. My understanding is that the child is just as autistic as pre-intervention! As already noted, autism is not behaviour. My worry is that the notion of changing autism, if that is what stems from the concept of this spectrum, is one that (1) will encourage parents to believe that their child could become 'less autistic', (2) indicates that being autistic in and of itself is inherently a bad thing and (3) causes all sorts of judgements on a child based on how that child behaves. To my mind, one's energy is far better directed at identifying what causes an autistic child anxiety or difficulty and addressing that, not attempting in some way to make a child somehow different from how he or she is naturally wired. I must be clear here – I am not for one moment suggesting that the very disabling impact that autism (plus environment) can have on some children does not need urgent attention. What I am suggesting is that this is down to a myriad of factors, not the 'severity' of autism.

Note on behaviour: autism is not behaviour. Therefore, somehow judging a person *only* by how she behaves is very unlikely to give anyone a true understanding of that person. Some autistic children will behave in all sorts of very 'autistically normal' ways that are deemed so out of line with PNT development that they are seen as problematic, when in fact one might have a perfectly happy child; alternatively, one might have a child who 'presents' at a behavioural level in the same way as his PNT peers but who might be going through enormous problems. Basing assumptions *only* on the presentation of a person is a dangerous game to play. (NB: I am not suggesting that understanding behaviour is not important – conversely, it is crucial. What I am suggesting is that only using the *presentation* of the child to make a decision regarding his or her *neurological* state may give spectacularly false impressions.)

My final rationale is that I simply cannot believe that there is some mythical continuum whereby one becomes less and less autistic and suddenly crosses over an invisible line to become non-autistic. If one *were* to ascribe to this concept, then surely a natural, logical argument would be that if one carried on along this continuum, way past the 'autism crossover line', then one would become more and more 'normal', as though there were some kind of absolute in terms of 'normality' – which I find very hard to believe! So my view is that, to best understand the child, we need to understand – on a day-to-day basis – just what impact being autistic has within that environment, and what we need to do to best support the child, both short and long term, taking those components into account. It's pretty simple as a concept – after all, it's what we would do as good parents for *all* children, the only difference being that, in the case of the autistic child, we need to understand (as best we can) the child's perspective through 'the autism lens' as opposed to anything else.

Myth: autistic traits (everyone is a bit autistic)

You may need to prepare yourself in life for people telling you, 'Oh, your child is autistic? I'm a bit like that, too.' My view is that this is as inane as a woman saying to a man, 'Oh, I'm a bit male too – because I've got two legs and two arms as well, so I have got male traits.' While I acknowledge that having two arms and two legs is *not* what characterizes 'maleness' (let's not go there), the point I am making is that if one accepts that there is *nothing* that an autistic person will display (in terms of traits and characteristics) that cannot be shared with a non-autistic person, the whole concept of traits rather falls apart. For example, lacking eye contact could be seen as an 'autistic trait', but do all autistic people lack eye contact? No. Is lacking eye contact unique to autistic people? Definitely not. So is lacking eye contact really an autistic trait? Even if 'trait' (which means 'distinguishing feature') were to be used in a much looser way – for example, 'something that is often found in the population' (in this case the autistic population) – then it still faces the same issues outlined above. Sharing a 'trait' – in this example, lacking eye contact – doesn't make you any more or less autistic than anything else. The reason behind your lack of eye contact is unlikely to be the same as for the autistic person.

Why is any of this an issue? Well, I think that going down the road of 'Well, we're all a bit like that' is to massively demean what it means to be autistic, almost as if it can be dismissed out of hand. It can also be extremely distressing for the autistic person, particularly someone struggling with a particular component of being autistic. It somehow lessens the autistic experience or makes it less valid, which is, to my mind, incredibly unfair and possibly detrimental to the well-being of the autistic person.

Myth: autistic children are unsociable

This one is easy! Being autistic – despite what popular media might depict – has nothing whatsoever to do with sociability. Sociability is the *desire* to engage at a social level, and there is just as much variance within the autistic population as there is within the PNT – in other words, one may find a highly sociable autistic child and a

PNT child who much prefers his or her own company, and/or vice versa.

What is far more important is to understand that the *desire* to socialize may not be apparent in a child for whom socializing is *difficult.* So if a child finds engaging with others difficult, he or she may choose not to do it; this should not be seen as a lack of desire or need.

Myth: autistics are savants

Some media representations are based on autistic children and adults having savant abilities. This is because, in the main, the purpose of the media is to sell – be it a book or film or magazine article. Savant abilities are in all probability something that can be used as part of a plot line or to engage an audience as an interesting 'story'. However, this has led to a misconception that *all* autistic folk have some kind of savant ability. The reality is that, while some may have savant abilities, the vast majority do not.

Myth: autistic children lack pretend play and are not imaginative

Many people still believe that children lack imaginative, pretend play – but while this might the case for some children, it is clearly not the case for others. Play is a very subjective thing anyway: PNT children have a massive range of preferences when it comes to play, so why shouldn't the same apply to autistic children? For some autistic children the whole notion of pretend is a nonsense, which is, strictly, extremely (autistically) logical. Why waste time pretending to be someone you're not? For some autistic people this would seem absolutely absurd, so it may not be the case that those children *cannot* pretend play in this way, but simply that they don't see the point.

Other kids may be brilliant at *demonstrating* pretend play but may not actually be particularly proficient at it, which may be misleading. It may be that they are copying (more on this in Chapter 5), which appears on the surface to be genuine pretence but in reality is simply a depiction of a scene in a favourite movie or something they have picked up on in nursery. Some children have astonishing memories and are able to act entire movies or TV programmes (or family interactions), to the point that it appears to be either excellent imaginative play or brilliant social interaction, when the reality is that it is actually fantastic copying behaviour.

Imagination, in my view, is far too vast simply to refer to as a concept – after all, there are all sorts of ways in which a child might (or might not) be imaginative. It is absolutely certain that some autistic children have incredible imaginations when it comes to – for example – creativity. Making up stories, acting them out, fantasy worlds – these may be part and parcel of the autistic child's life. Dare I suggest that some children who fit this description grow up to be very well-thought-of authors, playwrights and film directors?

Theory of mind

Theory of mind has been a dominant, popular theory for many years, but just because it's popular does not mean that it is any more (or less) important than other theories, nor does its popularity mean that it explains autism better than anything else.

Theory of mind, in brief, is the ability to 'see things from another's perspective' – metaphorically, 'to put oneself into someone else's shoes'. At its most basic, it involves having an understanding that what one thinks is *not* necessarily what everyone else thinks; at its most extreme it involves almost being a mind reader! The theory has been identified as possibly explaining autism, at least to a certain degree, in that a *lack* of theory of mind might explain some autistic experiences. In actual fact, in current academic circles, there is more of a leaning towards people believing that there is a *delay* in the acquisition of theory of mind, and/or possibly a *partial level* of theory of mind rather than a complete lack; however, I still suggest that the theory could be seen in a different context altogether anyway.

What theory of mind suggests is that people (in general) have the ability to intuitively empathize – in other words to see things and empathize with others from their perspective without consciously having to think about it or work it out. As regards autism theory, the basis is that a delayed theory of mind or a 'poor' theory of mind could explain, at least in part, the autistic experience. For example, if a child does not have an intuitive understanding of someone else's 'mind' then this may logically lead to being brutally honest – for example, giving an honest opinion of someone having put on weight. The rationale is that while this may be factually correct the child may not recognize that pointing it out might actually be hurtful to the person in question. However, as is so often the case in autism, it may be somewhat more complicated than that! Of course, such an exchange may indeed stem from a lack of intuitive empathy, but it may also stem from the logical perspective of an autistic person. After all, surely the overweight person in question is well aware of his own weight gain anyway, so what is the problem in articulating it? (See the example on p. 81 of Chapter 5.) This is an example, in fact, of how *illogical* the PNT might be perceived to be by the autistic population.

Going back to theory of mind, having a high degree of empathy may also lead to a higher skills level for deception, and it is often the case that autistic children are rather poor at deception and may more readily proffer 'truth' (from their perspective) and find it less easy to lie. Please do note, though, that the concept that autistic children never lie is an absolute nonsense – some may lie pretty well! It is, however, far more common to find that autistic children (and adults) find lying a difficult thing to do – and the concept of 'white lies' may be highly problematic as well, for the very reason outlined above!

My greatest criticism of theory of mind in relation to autism is not really based on the theory itself. We know full well that not all autistic children lack a theory of mind and that the theory does not explain autism in its entirety, but it may be useful in part to understand the autistic experience. My issue is more to do with the fact that autistic people are the ones who are branded as somehow inferior for lacking this theory of mind, when in fact the same could easily be said of the PNT. After all, how many PNTs can justifiably suggest that they have good empathic skills when it comes to understanding the autistic population?

My view is that the only 'fair' way to discuss theory of mind is to acknowledge that what we are actually referring to is what I term 'cross-neurological theory of mind', and that any issues with it work both ways – that is, while the autistic child may lack an understanding of the PNT brain, equally (or even more so) the PNT will lack an understanding of the autistic brain. The reason I suggest that the balance illustrates that the PNT are actually 'worse' at understanding the autistic brain is simply a matter of statistics. Because the autistic population is significantly in the minority, the emphasis is (usually) on them to align to the 'norm' of the society around them. This means that the pressure is on the autistic child to develop *learned* empathy – to have to consciously work things out from a PNT perspective in order to 'fit in'. This, I would argue, is only very rarely the case the other way around.

Just as an aside, but to make the point: if all PNTs did have a good autistic theory of mind, then books like this would never need to be written, autism conferences would cease to exist and I would be out of a job!

Myth: there is a 'normal' child locked inside somewhere, waiting to get out

Your child *is* normal – autistically normal, yes, but still absolutely normal for him or her. What is normal to one person will not be normal to another; we all have our own normal. Most of us are allowed to be ourselves, simply because there is usually an innate drive to behave and present in ways that do not make us stand out from the norm unless we choose to do so for a specific reason. Autistic children tend to be far less bothered about what other people think about them – in fact, I think it is often one of the most endearing characteristics so often found in children. It's not that they don't care per se, it's more a case that they don't care what the majority of people think, as they don't even know them! Logically, why would they be bothered what a stranger thinks about them?

What I really want to quash is the ridiculous notion that somehow there is an inner child 'locked away' inside this autistic 'shell' and that by 'breaking' the autistic shell one might release this other child, who will be so different from the original. I mean, just writing it down makes me feel somewhat strange – it is such an outdated and harmful notion I barely like to even think about it. So, just to be clear: the concept of there being some kind of duality and that autism is something that can be got rid of in order to release a 'normal' child is utter, complete, absolute nonsense. Rather than seeking to 'normalize' your child you are far better off getting to know her and understanding what makes her tick. This, in fact, may 'unlock' all sorts of connections – communication, sensory understanding, light-bulb moments when you finally realize what has been going on 'behind the scenes'. Clarity – over why your child is the way she is – and acceptance – of the notion of 'autistic normality' – will be a far more rewarding journey than trying (and failing) to change your child from who she is to someone whom she is not.

You can change all sorts of things about how a child will manage and interact with the world – what you are *not* doing is changing the child from being autistic to anything else at all.

Social skills and autistic sociality

Autistic children are deemed to be 'impaired in social skills'. OK, but in reality what they actually are at times is bemused by the somewhat bizarre (to them) social interaction of the PNT and, thus, they possibly lack *PNT social skills*. This is not the same as suggesting that autistic people are impaired in social skills per se.

Take a bit of time to listen in to social conversations, just to get a bit of awareness as to what content they have. Similarly, reflecting on PNT social interaction and then re-looking at it from an autism perspective can be extremely illuminating. From an autistically logical perspective PNT social interaction can be seriously odd! Consider the following social comments followed by autistically logical inner responses.

- *'Good morning!'* What do you mean by this? How would you know whether my morning is any good – and this is not even taking into account that it's 9 a.m. and I've only been up since 7.15 a.m., so the vast majority of the morning is yet to come. Can you now see not just into the future but into *my* future? You don't look particularly happy, so I'm not even convinced that you really mean it's a particularly good morning. Anyway, haven't you heard the news? There's all sorts of stuff going on in the world that mean I wouldn't classify this morning anywhere near the realm of 'good'. Would you like to rethink now?

- *'Hi mate, how are you feeling?'* I am not your mate. In animalistic terms I am most definitely not coupled with you, nor do I intend to be. In social terms I dislike you, and seeing as 'mates' are supposed to like one another I fail to see how this 'greeting' or question is valid in any sense. However, I am not feeling at all good – I had a terrible night's sleep and my piles are playing up. I dislike all of these people I have to work with and am literally counting down the minutes until I can escape. However, as I recall, the last time I gave an honest answer to your line of enquiry I got disciplined, so I shall breathe an inner sigh, grit my teeth and copy you lot by replying with the lie 'All right'.

- *'It's cold today!'* I have no idea how to respond to this inanity. Coldness is clearly relative, but that aside, seeing as we are sharing the same vicinity and have been outside in a similar proximity to one another, we are presumably both well aware of the air temperature. Quite why you feel the need to explain something that is self-evident I have no idea. Perhaps you think I have some hitherto unknown condition that makes me unaware of coldness – I don't know. In the meantime, I think it's safest simply to ignore you.

- *'Did you see that programme last night . . .?'* Yes, I did. However, past experience tells me that whether I saw it or not, you will regale me with repetition as regards the programme itself. Since I have already seen it this is completely illogical to me. Please go away.

These are rather 'tongue-in-cheek' examples but they do give an insight into how, from a certain perspective, social engagement might be viewed. There are all sorts of reasons why PNT people interact at a social level, but not all of these reasons will be applicable to the autistic individual. Therefore, not all autistic children will develop these 'skills' within the social arena as part of their natural development.

Of course, the converse to suggesting that autistics are poor at PNT social skills is equally the case – the PNT in the main make for terrible social autistics! Show me an average PNT who has well-developed autistic social skills and I'll give you a medal. And yet the PNT are not labelled as impaired in (autistic) social skills, despite the fact that sitting enjoying company in total silence can be highly logical, immensely satisfying and deeply enjoyable. The removal of 'small talk' can be the most glorious blessing, allowing people to have a sensible conversation without the litter of erroneous communications that bear no relevance to the subject matter. Again, the list could go on.

I am absolutely convinced that there is such a thing as 'autistic sociality' (and a very clear 'nod' here to Dr Joanna Baker-Rogers, whose PhD thesis covers this area very well). Autistic sociality is that which pertains to how an autistic child might engage *at a social level* either with other autistic children or with a well-trained PNT! As noted, autistic children may well demonstrate autistic social skills – which are rarely found in the PNT population. Yet again, the impairment-based model seems actually to simply be judging a population for being in the minority as opposed to having any real merit.

Social hangovers

Being in a non-autistic friendly social environment – even fleetingly – can have a huge impact on the autistic child. Having to 'act' as a social being outside the natural order of things – in other words, what society expects of the autistic child much of the time – can be massively energy-consuming at both an intellectual and an emotional level (more on this in later chapters). It's worth just noting here that the concept of a 'social hangover' – in other words, needing a (sometimes considerable) time to recover – may be requisite for the autistic individual following social engagement, however brief or innocuous that interaction might seem to you. Never underestimate the energy required in many cases for the autistic child! And never underestimate the duration that may be required before the child is able to re-engage after a social hangover.

Spiky profiles

One of the important concepts related to autism that is clearly the case for most, if not all, children is that of the spiky profile. What this means is that autistic children are highly likely to demonstrate strengths and weaknesses at much more obvious degrees than the PNT. Everyone will have strengths and weaknesses, of course, but these tend to be acutely more obvious within the autistic population. This goes well beyond academic subjects – it can cover all or any 'skill' set – as well as what are deemed developmental milestones. In other words, there is little point making any assumptions of skill based on any other particular strength. One good example of this is verbal communication. The PNT in the main tend to have very similar skills in expressive and receptive verbal communication, so their ability to talk at any given level is usually very similar to the level at which they can understand spoken language. This is not an assumption that can be made for the autistic child, who may be non-verbal with excellent communication or have excellent expressive language with difficulties in understanding others' spoken word.

This spiky profile is essential to understand, otherwise all sorts of incorrect assumptions might be made. Comments such as 'Well, she *must* be able to do X because she can do Y' should be taken with extreme caution! It is not 'autistically logical' to assume that a well-honed skill in one area will mean that skills in others are equally as well honed; while it may often be the case for the PNT, it is not usually the case for the autistic child. For example, being a brilliant orator at a conference does not mean one is any good at social chit-chat, and the further examples one could give here are infinite!

4

Sensory profiles

Why are sensory profiles important?

So sensory 'issues' are being recognized more and more as part of the autistic experience. I put 'issues' in inverted commas deliberately; as is so often the case when it comes to autism, the seemingly immediate direction of travel is one of negativity! DSM-5[1], for example, cites hyper- or hyporeactivity to sensory input as part of the criteria for autism, as well as:

> unusual interests in sensory aspects of the environment (e.g. apparent indifference to pain/temperature, adverse response to specific sounds or textures, excessive smelling or touching of objects, visual fascination with lights or movement).

It may not seem too bad on first reading, but the tone is still pejorative – 'unusual', 'indifference', 'adverse' are all rather negative terms. While it is crystal-clear that some sensory experiences can be overwhelmingly negative, many may have the opposite impact. Indeed, reading autobiographical accounts and blogs and chatting to people can give you a sense of some of the extremely positive, pleasurable sensory experiences that some autistic people have.

When it comes to understanding your child, having as good an understanding of the sensory experience as possible is absolutely vital. While various theories try to explain autism, as noted in Chapter 3, none of them does so very well. One of the often-missed areas of autism life is the whole sensory domain – and yet the impact it can have on the autistic child is immense. You may find that, actually, the sensory processing of your child explains more about his or her way of being than many other theories.

---

[1] 2013, APA.

I have written much of this chapter from the first person – little stories, in a sense. This is partly because obviously one's sensory experience is deeply personal, but it also allows me to 'bring to life' the very real experiences that some autistic people articulate. Before I start on that section, though, here is some of the theory behind sensory perception from an autistic perspective.

Over- and undersensory responses

In a nutshell, autistic people may experience any one (or more) of the five primary senses either in a *more* sensitive manner than the PNT or in a *less* sensitive manner than the PNT. I am only 'comparing' in this instance to demonstrate that the actual lived experience for the autistic child may be (hugely) different in comparison to the PNT – this doesn't make it 'right' or 'wrong' but it does make it very different. This is an area that many PNTs find very difficult to understand at an empathic level, yet all people will have their own way of perceiving reality, irrespective of whether they are autistic or not. What is important – or, rather, *essential* – is that there is an understanding that those differences exist and they are taken extremely seriously. Here are some key 'rules' for thinking about sensory experiences.

- Believe the autistic person when he tells you how he is experiencing sensory input. However improbable, however vastly different from anything you might perceive this may be, it is absolutely clear that many autistic people process senses very differently from the PNT.
- Take sensory experiences very seriously. Ignoring the negative impact of the sensory environment is, simply, very poor practice. It is vital that all sensory environments are as friendly as possible for your autistic child. This is not always practically possible, of course, but it remains just as important!
- Understand and accept that reactions to sensory environments are not necessarily predictable. However hard one tries, there may be something you have not considered!

There are other critical issues that also need to be taken into account, including the following.

- Sensory experiences may change – the child may react differently *to the same sensory environment* from one moment to the next. This can literally be within minutes; further explanation to follow!

- Sensory profiles will very probably change over time, sometimes dramatically. It may be that one specific sensory characteristic might simply disappear overnight; for example, your child may be intolerant to the noise of the vacuum cleaner one day, and all of a sudden this is no longer a problem. It is essential, though, to recognize that while the child may no longer have a problem, it does not detract from the very real sensitivity previously shown.
- A child is likely to be *both* hyper- and hyposensitive to sensory information, sometimes even within the same sense! While this may sound odd or unusual, rest assured it is perfectly 'autistically normal'.
- Just because a child demonstrates a particular sensitivity in one domain, it does not mean that one can automatically assume that the sensitivity will be demonstrated across environments. So, for example, a child may be apparently very sensitive to noise, but noise in one environment may not be tolerated while noise in another may be perfectly acceptable.
- Synaesthesia[2] is very real despite sounding improbable.
- Perceptual reality is exactly that – real. For the person experiencing the world it is their reality, however different it might be from yours, and thus it should be taken extremely seriously. 'Perceptual reality' is the phrase that I use to mean what the person is experiencing in a sensory manner; each person will have his or her own perceptual reality, and those experiences, even within the same environment, can differ hugely between the PNT and the autistic child, and between one autistic child and the next. So if there are three children in the same environment, one PNT and two autistic children, each perceptual reality could be vastly different between all three children, and each is absolutely 'real' to that individual child.

So what does all this mean in reality? We have five primary senses, which may be impacted in various ways:

- hearing (auditory)
- seeing (visual)

---

[2] Synaesthesia: one sense is processed as another, e.g. 'seeing' colour, or 'feeling' words.

- tasting (gustatory)
- feeling (tactile)
- smelling (olfactory).

Each of these may differ for the autistic child in comparison to the PNT range of sensitivity. However, there are also two other (main) areas in which an autistic child may differ: vestibular and proprioception. Vestibular is, basically, balance and movement and related activity. Proprioception is about one's sense of self in relation to one's own body and the surrounding area. As with the five primary senses, vestibular and proprioception may also be either hyper- or hyposensitive for the autistic child and, as with the five primary senses, can explain a lot about why a child might react in a certain way within a specific environment.

Why does sensory impact change?

The impact of the environment can differ, sometimes massively, from one minute to the next, one day to the next, one week to the next, one year to the next – and so on. There may be several explanations for this, but the main ones are these.

- The environment itself *is* actually different so the perceptual reality of the child differs – it may be that the PNT adult might not appreciate or pick up on the difference, but it is there!
- The child's general well-being will impact massively on his or her tolerance levels to the sensory environment. Well-being will include: anxiety levels, stress levels, physical well-being, how rested the child is, emotional stability – the list could go on. The important thing to note is that the less 'well' the child is, the more likely it is that the sensory environment will adversely impact on the child.

Conversations between you and your child

How this is set out: some questions are posed by a parent and answered by a child, and then the next question is a different parent and thus a different child. There are some sections that involve longer conversations with the same child – it should be obvious!

I was wondering, why will you wear that jumper and not this one?

Do you not realize the two are so completely different? OK, let me explain. They do look the same, I'll grant you that. But the one I can tolerate has been washed more times, so the texture is – to me, anyway – absolutely different. This one makes me feel all snuggly and fuzzy (in a good way) while that one makes my skin crawl! And before you think you can go and simply wash that one a few times, think again. I know for a fact that we have changed washing powders, so the effects will be different. Just let me wear this one and don't worry about diverse jumper wearing – it's over-rated!

Seriously, what is wrong with T-shirts?

Nothing – nothing at all. But why would I wear a short-sleeved top when I can wear a long-sleeved one? It's my proprioception, you see – I struggle to know where the ends of my arms are unless I've got something else physical that isn't a part of me to gauge arm length. It's lush when I've got a long-sleeved top with nice tight cuffs – I know exactly where my arms are at all times!

Seriously, why do you wear nothing but T-shirts?

Isn't it obvious? It's because I have sensory sensitivity on my arms, so anything touching them causes major discomfort. It literally feels as though I have ants crawling over my skin, so please don't insist on long sleeves – it is actually unbelievably stressful. When I'm forced to wear long sleeves I can't concentrate on anything else, so it really disrupts my day. I can't concentrate at school, in fact it even impacts on my ability to speak – so T-shirt it is for me, please!

But surely you'll freeze to death?

Nah, I'm totally OK with wearing a T-shirt even when it's cold. My temperature control is different from yours, that's all. It's like that for a lot of us autistics. My mate is the opposite to me – she wears several layers even in the heat, she loves it!

You simply refuse to wear that particular top. What's the problem with it?

It sounds so stereotypical, but it's the label! If you don't take the label out it's all I can feel when I wear that top – it's unbelievably distracting. And don't think that cutting the label out is OK. If anything, it's worse – the label then becomes sharp! Unstitching it completely is the safest way to go, I reckon.

OK, so that's your top sorted. What about these socks?

Well, with my tops it's the label, with the socks it's the seam – simply horrible! It feels so clunky and uncomfortable. The only way I will wear those socks is if I make sure that the bulky seam is lined up exactly so the pressure on each of my toes is just the same – which, as we know, takes ages and you get annoyed that I'm taking 20 minutes per sock to put them on! But that time when you tried to put the socks on me without making sure the seams were lined up, remember? I was screaming all day and you just didn't understand why! Sometimes I can get away with turning them inside out so the seams are on the outside; it's better, but still not brilliant. What is brilliant is when you buy me seamless socks – now they are pure joy to wear! Other things to take note: socks that are just a little too tight or just a little too loose – both are intolerable. I promise I'm not being fussy – wearing those kinds of socks makes me feel I just can't balance properly, I feel wobbly all the time – it's horrible, and actually quite scary!

I had no idea – is there anything else related to clothes that I need to understand?

Oh yes, loads, probably. It's funny though – for each of my preferences about clothes I know others who seem to be the opposite. So I love my really tight clothes, the ones that make me feel in a cocoon, all safe and snuggly. My mate, though, he hates that and loves really loose, baggy clothing – personally, I have no idea how he can cope with it, but each to their own. I do know a girl, though – she seriously stresses over clothes that are a certain colour. Some colours seem to bother her more than others, but she does tell me that the worst colours actually hurt her eyes. She used to get so stressed because she thought everyone must know and that they were deliberately exposing her to pain – it was only when she got chatting to her dad about it that she realized that painful eyes in response to colour wasn't everyone's experience. She's tons better now. Even when she has to go out and so doesn't have any control over what people are wearing, she takes really dark sunglasses and pops them on – it really helps, so she tells me.

You know sometimes the clothes themselves, as such, are not the problem. I love the smell of washing powder, for example, but clothes that have just come out of the wash are simply far too overwhelming to put on straightaway – I need a good few days before the smell is 'quiet' enough for me to wear them comfortably. Other things are the type of buttons or even the noise of the zip – these are the sorts of things that help me decide what I can wear and what I can't.

One last thing: I'm not saying it's that common but I have noticed a few of my autistic friends only ever wearing shorts. When I ask them about it, they tell me that the feeling of trousers (usually against their knees) is literally intolerable. In fact, one guy told me that the feeling was one of intense pain; as soon as he had the choice he took to wearing shorts to alleviate the pain. I felt so bad for his parents who genuinely hadn't known and dressed the poor chap in trousers for years. He was non-verbal at the time and couldn't communicate his distress. I don't know who ended up more traumatized by the whole thing, him or his parents! It just goes to show, though, how important it is for parents to understand our sensory needs.

You know, one thing I have noticed and would love to know more about: you seem to approach hugging in a very different way from your brother – am I right?

Yeah, I'm sure you are. You see, for me, hugging is fantastic in some ways but fraught with danger at the same time. So I am wary, at the very least. I've chatted to my mates about this and they all seem to view hugging in slightly different ways, so I will pass on my thoughts and also what they've said to me. You can then make your own mind up!

For me, full-on 'frontal' hugging is simply too overwhelming, which is why I do that kind of sidling upside-down squashy thing –

my version of a hug! And it has to come from me to instigate it – if someone were to try and hug me unawares, I would seriously have a meltdown! I am pretty sure that I'm person-intolerant, in that contact with people needs to be kept to a minimum unless it's someone I know really well and feel uber-comfy with. Mostly, the discomfort of physical contact is enough for me to opt out – it doesn't mean I'm unkind or don't care, I promise! I was thinking about it the other day, and decided that it's the combination of touch, smell (people can smell really, really offensive to me without meaning to!) and predictability – each of those things is so important to me, so the combination is usually enough to put me off. Try not to judge me – when I do have contact with you, however minimal, it means I am showing you tons of affection, similar to those bear hugs you get from my favourite brother.

I do know folk who are more into hugging than me but they still have stipulations. Some only like really hard, tight, squeezy hugs so they can barely breathe, while others need hugs to be so light touch it hardly seems like a hug at all! Some will readily hug others (be the 'hugger') but won't like it if they are hugged back (being the 'huggee'). And, of course, it should go without saying that hugging should not be accompanied with things like face-grabbing or arm squeezing – these are in a different tolerance zone altogether! Oh, and do remember that if we are to be involved in this hugging lark, please don't be expecting us to chatter at the same time – one thing at a time, please!

By the way, it just reminded me: those people who love really hard hugs, they do tell me that deep pressure in all sorts of ways is a sublime experience. Some even report that it massively reduces their stress levels. I know kids who love their weighted blankets at bedtime, for example, and all sorts of activities that 'allow' them to engage with deep pressure.

So you're saying that there might be a preference for light touch or hard, is that right?

Oh yes, definitely. Mind you, it can be that some people love light touch in some ways and hard touch in others – very confusing, I know! But me, for example – I only really like touch that is in my control, otherwise I get very twitchy indeed. It goes beyond just light and hard – it might include, for example, what is touching what. I do know of a young lady who simply cannot bear any person touching her bare skin unless she knows them really well. It's so fascinating – she tells me that the more she gets to know someone and the more relaxed she is around that person, the less unpleasant direct skin contact is. But if a stranger were to touch her – even accidentally, like walking past her on the street – it can be so bad it's similar to being hit! I know others for whom light touch itself – irrespective of whether that's skin contact or otherwise – is simply pure pain; it's often those who find very firm contact so much easier to 'digest' (but, of course, not always).

Another thing to consider is where the actual touch is directed. I'm pretty cool with a head massage, for example. In fact, I love them – really sends me into a trance and I feel as if I'm floating. It's fantastic that you book me in each week; it's one of the things I look forward to the most! But I do know some people who would absolutely go into meltdown if anyone went anywhere near their hair.

I'm sorry – *what?* Autistic people don't like their hair being touched?

No, that's far too general. But for those who might be termed 'hair touch intolerant' it's a massive, massive deal. I've heard people say that the way in which they experience their hair being touched is akin to very real pain. For some, it's any kind of touch; for others, it might be hair-washing, brushing, combing; and for a few having a haircut is literally agony. It sounds pretty extreme, I know, but for some people it's their reality.

I had no idea – what should we do about it?

Well, there are a few things that seem to work for some people. I know there are products out there that can be used to clean hair without getting it wet, which can be a brilliant outcome for some of my friends. The hair-cutting is a major issue – I know someone who can have a haircut but only with electric clippers, not with scissors – but, mostly, the people I talk to just ask to have long hair!

Actually, while I'm on this subject, there are parallels with cutting nails. You know how I used to hate having my nails cut? It's because it was so uncomfortable, bordering on painful. Now that you let me soak myself in the bath for an hour before having them cut, it's OK. My mate used to be similar. In his case, though, his mum found that using a nail file as part of his evening routine worked a treat – literally a few seconds of filing every night meant that the monthly stress of actual nail-cutting was cut out. Mind you, they did learn the hard way that it is essential to use a specific type of nail file; in his case it was the nail boards that aren't made of metal that suited him.

So cutting hair and nails can actually be painful?

Oh yes, definitely. In fact, pain is another thing that can be so hard for some people to understand – sometimes I think they should forget about trying to understand it and simply accept it for what it is.

What do you mean? Can you give any examples?

Definitely! Some of it is hypersensitivity, some of it is synaesthesia, some a combination of both. Of course, then there's hyposensitivity to pain that people find equally difficult to accept!

OK, so some real-life examples. I've already told you about how some people find it painful to have their hair or nails cut. And there was the colour pain I mentioned earlier. All of these are examples that people might think we are making up, but we really aren't. Sometimes, though, like the colour example, it's not even touch that is painful – some noises can be painful, as can some smells or tastes. Conversely, I do know some kids who have seemingly really hurt themselves – like falling out of a tree and ending up in hospital with a cast – but at the time didn't seem in the slightest bit bothered. And yet that same kid could get really distressed about what others might not even notice, like his watch strap being ever so slightly too tight!

The light touch thing can also be a major problem for some, light touch being processed as actual pain. There are some kids who need to wear really bulky clothes or several layers to 'protect' them from people brushing past them in the street or in the corridor at school. You can even go online to find undergarments that will help for kids who are really hypersensitive in this way.

Can you explain why you went through that phase of not brushing your teeth?

There are so many things that can have an impact on the whole teeth-brushing experience! For example, all of the following could make or break teeth time:

- the taste of the toothpaste;
- the colour of the toothpaste;
- the smell of the toothpaste;
- the brush itself – manual or electric, the texture of the bristles, the colour of the handle . . .;
- if it's an electric toothbrush, the noise and feel of vibrations – these are crucial;
- water temperature;
- the sound of the water running in the sink;
- the proximity of you standing next to me;
- the fact that you are looking right at me, which makes me feel stressed;
- not knowing how long I should brush my teeth for, so feeling that it's best simply not to start (when you gave me that timer it really helped);
- having to brush my teeth when I have only recently eaten;
- being told I need to hurry up – if I'm rushed I tend to freeze!

So all those reasons were important to me, and getting the combination of them with the 'correct' permutations took some time – but it was worth it in the end. Mind you, most of my mates have a totally different list!

Your older sister is really strict about where she sits in class at school. Do you know why this might be?

Well, she's not spoken to me about it. I don't like thinking about what school might be like, but knowing what I know about her I reckon I could make a pretty good guess. First of all, she will need to be at the front of the class – she would hate all the visual stimulation of having to see across everyone else. Funnily enough, I know some people for whom this would be their worst nightmare and who would choose to sit at the back – they are the ones who hate being in the spotlight and don't want to feel everyone looking at them if they were sitting at the front. Anyway, she would also want to sit at the end of a row, so she feels she can escape when need be. She would prefer no one to sit next to her so she didn't have to tolerate the proximity of another person – this will be because she would find someone's smell bothersome, and any noises made by the other person would drown out the teacher. And she would want to be at the right-hand side of the class. No idea why, but she always likes to be on the right-hand side of everything – sitting in the car, walking, whatever. She says it's something to do with visually balancing things out!

She's just one person, though. Some people might be affected by other things, like the noise of the clock, whether they can see out of a window or the sunlight being in their eyes or how easily they can see the door. There are so many different reasons for something as simple as where to sit, but it can be so important too!

I have never, ever known anyone to be so fussy about choosing and wearing new shoes. Why can't you enjoy buying new things the same as other kids?

I'm not 'fussy', I promise! I know what I can tolerate and what I can't, that's all. And I do mean 'tolerate' – you see, many of the shoes I have to try on are painful. So even going shopping for new shoes is an experience that I absolutely dread. I know it takes ages – trust me, it might seem like a real drag for you, but just imagine being me! I hate the whole thing, and as most of the shoes that are forced on to me hurt me the whole day is an endless parade of pain – with very little gain, it seems to me! I don't like meeting new people, I absolutely hate my very sensitive feet being touched and I cannot bear the very hard edges that new shoes almost always have. Shoe shopping includes all three of these things, countless times. Is it any wonder that I don't like it? I sometimes wonder if it might be better thinking ahead; if I find a pair of shoes that I can tolerate, and we all know how much I like routine and similarity, why couldn't we just buy several pairs of the same kind of shoe in different sizes? That way I'm happy and you don't have the awful experience of dragging me around for the day, probably seeming like a terribly ungrateful child – which I'm really not!

It's similar when you take me shopping for clothes in general, by the way. I don't like bright lights, I don't like crowds, I don't like all the weird smells that are in lots of these shops – and I absolutely detest having to go into the changing rooms, not knowing who has been there before me. It would be so much less painful for me to be allowed to shop on the internet or for you to shop on my behalf – you know what I like and don't like, you're a great parent. I really don't mind if you fill my wardrobe with very similar clothes – in fact it's quite a comfort!

Fair enough!

But, staying on the theme of fussiness, why do you insist on eating the way you do?

Eating can be a real chore for me. Sometimes it is the texture of the food that I simply cannot tolerate – it's painful in my mouth and makes me gag. I know some people who are similar to me as well, but they like really soft, mushy food whereas I love mine as hard as possible so my mouth knows exactly what's in it and I can enjoy the breakdown from hard, solid food to the consistency for it being swallowed.

I also hate different foods touching each other on the plate – it's just so wrong! Actually, I am more tolerant than some. My friend likes her food on separate plates, a bit like an everyday tapas; each type of food has its own little plate so she can easily see the difference and choose what to have and when, without any cross-contamination (as she calls it) – actually, come to think of it, I quite like that idea myself!

Some autistic kids can only eat really bland food and others are at the other end of the scale, noshing down on extreme-tasting curries and the like. Our taste buds are the same as our other senses, I reckon – either over- or undersensitive, hence the preference for certain types of food. It's no big deal – so long as we get the right nutrition, we're pretty happy with a fairly limited diet. It seems odd to us – as kids you grown-ups seem to want us to eat this massive range of food, but I can see so many adults who only really eat a very limited number of dinners each week. Strange, that.

I also know of some kids who are really funny about the colour of their food. They tell me that they can taste the colour but not the actual taste, if that makes sense. Pretty cool – but again, the grown-ups seem to either not believe them or think it's some kind of fad. It really isn't, though. It reminds me of someone I met on autism camp who only ate food of a certain shape. He found it really difficult to eat anything with sharp edges, as the sensation was as if his mouth was being cut. So he loved round things, or things like mash, which isn't 'sharp'.

Another kid has this amazing sense of taste, as if he knows what he likes and won't eat anything else, even if it is supposedly 'the same'. So he will only eat a certain brand of crisps. He knows full well if they are the same flavour but a different brand – I've seen him do a 'blind taste' and he gets it right every time!

I've noticed something you might be able to help with: you clap your hands over your ears and sometimes I think I know why (like when the dog barks), but other times, I really can't work out why

Really? I had no idea! So you can't hear the things I can? I have certain types of noises that pain my ears, and trying to block the sounds out means it's less painful. Yes, the dog barking is one of them – but have you noticed that certain dogs can bark and I'm OK with it while others are a different story? You see, my hearing is so sensitive, my ears will differentiate between what you might regard as tiny changes in sound. For example, I can quite happily listen to my teacher's voice at school when we are in the classroom, but when we are in the gym it's impossible to hear him. The sound is completely different!

Anyway, going back to other sounds I can't bear – sirens are one, and apparently I can hear them when you can't. I'd never realized that my hearing was so acute, but I guess it makes sense.

So, does hearing cause you other problems?

Loads! Well, some – but there are examples I could give, not just for me but also for others I know. Let me list some of them for you.

- There's this one kid who cannot hear anything at all unless it's the only noise in the room – she finds it impossible, for example, to hear her parents talking to her if the TV is on, nor can she hear the TV if her parents are chatting! It has to be one or the other.

- My mate literally lives in fear of certain noises. I've pointed out that sirens are a problem for me, which they are, but I can just about cope – he, on the other hand, used to refuse even to go out in case he heard certain sounds, that's how painful things are for him; he will go out now, though, now that he's allowed to wear his ear defenders. Have you seen them? I know autistic grown-ups that carry them about too, which is so cool. They simply pop them on when the noise around them gets too much. I wish all us kids were allowed them too, it would be a great way to self-regulate. Actually, I borrowed some once, and the funny thing was that as I knew I could use them whenever I wanted, it actually meant that I needed them less!

- Voices can be a real problem – when more than one person is speaking sometimes all the words get jumbled up together and make no sense at all; it's one of the reasons we prefer visual forms of communication, I reckon.

- This one isn't a problem – well, it can be, but it shouldn't be in my view! Some noises are so utterly delicious I could spend all day seeking them out and listening to them. They can be anything at all, ranging from certain words that rhyme to the noise of the cat sneezing. The point is, when I hear them I can almost melt into them, they are so incredible. The problem is when I get told to stop playing my recordings over and over again. I think it annoys other people, I don't see why else it would be a problem. I can listen to them for ages, and it's one of the most lush things I ever get to do.

- I do know one guy who doesn't even hear certain sounds, he sees them instead – literally. Like, if there is a banging noise, he sees flashes of light of certain colours. It's so fascinating – and the funny thing is, he didn't know that this was different from anyone else, it was purely by chance that he found out. I suppose it's a bit like being colour blind – how would you know if you were any different from anyone else?

I remember reading about this autistic person who could smell things from so far away, it seemed almost impossible. Have you heard of that?

Yes, sure. It's not actually that uncommon with me and my friends. Most of us have something or other going on with our sense of smell. Do you remember, for example, that time I really offended your mum because I told her she smelled too much? She thought I was being rude; I wasn't at all, it's just she had perfume on and my sense of smell is quite sensitive. It was just totally overwhelming; there was no way I could go near her. Lots of people don't realize the impact of wearing perfume or hair products or strong-smelling deodorant. For many of us it's too smelly – not necessarily bad, just too much altogether.

I also heard about someone who kept getting out of the pool – can you shed any light on that?

Yes, I heard about that. It was because the young man had a total intolerance of a certain type of perfume and he could smell it in the water if someone had been in who had been wearing it. He's so sensitive that if a woman wearing it got in at one end then, within seconds, he would be getting out from the other end, refusing to get back in!

This olfactory sensitivity sounds a bit extreme to me. Are you sure it's real?

Oh yes, for sure. You would be amazed at the things some autistic kids (and adults) can pick up. I know people who will sniff another person and recognize who they are just from their unique smell, for example.

But why would they need to do that?

I reckon the *need* to do it stems from a lack of ability to recognize faces very well. Some people call it face blindness – or prosopagnosia – and it literally means that people don't recall facial features so don't recognize people (in the conventional sense). Some autistic folk then work out ways for themselves as to how they might recognize a person, and sometimes that is via smell. Mind you, some people choose to focus on key features such as hair, which can be a bit of an issue when someone gets a haircut or even goes and dyes it! It can be a real problem for some people who are deemed really rude, just because they don't recognize someone – it's not like it's on purpose! I even know some adults who struggle to recognize their own kids or their spouse – it's nothing to do with not caring, though!

I've noticed that you squint sometimes. Do you know you're doing it?

Oh yes, I definitely know I'm doing it. It's because I can get really overwhelmed by all the visual information coming my way. It's as if there is no filter in my vision – everything my eyes pick up goes straight into my brain. I was chatting about this with one of my PNT mates; her brain only picks up on a fraction of what her eyes can pick up, so she can focus on what she needs to see. I'm very different: I have to physically narrow my field of vision so I can actually see things rather than everything being a massive blur of visual information.

You seem to notice patterns – is that correct?

Patterns are amazing – sometimes it's how I make sense of the world around me, and I adore the repetition and consistency of patterns. Patterns can be seen all over the place, if you know where to look! So, for example, I might develop a numerical pattern and count off certain types of cars in sequence; or there may be a visual pattern in the leaves of a tree which I can discern. Nature has tons of patterns and makes for very interesting viewing, sometimes to the point where I am unable to hear what you're saying as I'm so interested in the patterns!

It's similar – not exactly the same, but similar – to autistic kids who can see incredible detail in certain visual components of the world. So they might notice in an instant something of interest to them that remains 'hidden' to the rest of the population (unless you proactively point it out). Those kids can be a wealth of information in some areas, but because all their focus is taken up by things of interest to them, they might not pick up on the things that most people take for granted. Sometimes this means they might even miss out on things that most people would recognize as objects of danger, which can obviously be a worry for parents. They might need very specific teaching to work out what they need to look for in their environment to keep them safe.

**When you were younger, you spent ages lining things up –
like your toys – rather than playing with them. Why?**

I don't agree: I *was* playing with them! Just because I didn't (or
don't) 'play' in the same way as other kids doesn't make it any
less fun. I used to love the order of lining things up; it was visually pleasing and satisfying in ways that other kinds of play simply
don't achieve. In a similar way, I still love things being aligned 'correctly' – it offends my vision if things are not straight or parallel or
at precise right angles. When everything is correct and accounted
for I can relax and enjoy myself; until then, I'm on a mission to get
it right! I find it so difficult to understand why so few other people
are bothered in the same way, to be honest!

**Why won't you enter a supermarket with me? You get
seriously stressed and I just don't know why!**

It's a sensory thing. Loads of my mates are similar, but not always
for exactly the same reason. Basically, most supermarkets are hugely
sensory environments – by which I mean they are an absolute sense
sensation, with just so much going on that even the thought of
them makes me feel a bit wobbly. Next time you go in (leaving me
at home, please) just take a moment to identify everything that's
going on – the sights, smells, noise, changes in temperature, all the
different colours, an absolute bombardment of sensory information.
Seriously, I don't know how you cope with it! And this is before you
introduce all the trolleys, the people, the loudspeaker announce-
ments. Honestly, I sometimes wonder whether someone invented
supermarkets specifically thinking of how autism-unfriendly they
could possibly make them! For me it's the lighting – any fluorescent
lighting is bad for me (I can see the lights flicker and hear them
tick) so supermarkets with their abundance of the awful things
cause me to have serious brain ache. In fact, anywhere with those
lights causes me massive discomfort, which is something I worry
about for the future, seeing as so many big buildings have them.
Those energy-saving bulbs have a similar effect.

There are other reasons for other kids. Some don't like the disrup-
tion to neat, fully stocked shelves, for example. Others are OK until
someone decides to move the bread aisle and then it's a disaster!

I was on social media the other day and came across this weird phrase, 'happy flapping'. I haven't a clue what it means, have you?

Happy flapping – it's an autistic thing, we love a bit of happy flapping. Not so keen on the other kind though, the stressy worried flapping. We often flap at times of high emotional states, so happy flapping is exactly that, an expression of just how happy we are! It's basically a form of communication – lots of non-verbal kids do it and it can be invaluable to understand the meaning behind it so parents and teachers and suchlike can communicate effectively with the child. I did hear of a poor kid who kept being told to stop flapping – her teachers told her to sit on her hands instead. As it was her only form of communication it seemed pretty harsh to me, and I know for a fact it was extremely stressful for her. We do know that there is a time and a place but, really, communication is so important to us that we need all the understanding we can get! I once watched an autism conference online and it was full of autistic adults; instead of clapping when they heard a good speech they quietly flapped hands instead, it was one of the coolest things I've ever seen.

So is this flapping linked in with rocking at all?

Rocking is all about vestibular movement. Some of us have undersensitive vestibular systems, so we need to counterbalance it by rocking or swaying or any other kind of rhythmical movement. The need to do it, a bit like flapping, increases if we are under stress – in fact, it can be a great way to relieve stress. Again, being told to keep still is so hard: it's a bit like being told that you're not allowed to hold the handrail on a wobbly rope bridge. The feeling is one of being really unsteady and about to fall over at any time.

My friend works in a school for autistic children. She says she keeps losing a child and whenever they find him he's tucked away somewhere like the stationery cupboard!

Sounds pretty normal to me. Tons of us love small, enclosed spaces where we can feel really safe. In fact, sometimes open spaces can be incredibly disorientating, especially if we are not up against a wall.

Being in the middle of a wide open space can sometimes make me feel as if I'm drowning, I desperately need something tangible to hold on to, otherwise it really makes me panic. I wonder if your friend's chap at school is similar – it sounds like it to me. Talking of stationery cupboards, how about this for an example of good autism practice: I know an autistic adult who works in one! It's her own little office space now, without a telephone.

What does a telephone have to do with it?

Well, phones make awful noises when they ring and they are – by definition – absolutely unpredictable, so you're either in a mild state of panic (oxymoron, I know!), knowing that it might 'go off' at any point or you're having to cringe at the horrible noise it makes – or, almost worst of all, you have to be answering it, not knowing who will be on the other end nor what someone might ask of you! All in all, a telephone-free environment can suit some of us mightily well. In fact, one of the best things about mobile phones is the 'silent' option, and the fact that you can use it for texting or similar rather than actual speaking – very autism-friendly, I have to say!

5

Anxiety

What is anxiety?

Autism is frequently (almost always) associated with anxiety.[1] However, being autistic does *not* mean that a child will, *by definition*, be anxious. In other words, being autistic does not mean that one will be anxious all of the time, and there are some people who are clearly autistic who do not suffer from anxiety. Taking this into account, it stands to reason that, while autism and anxiety are linked – as there is clearly a much higher rate of anxiety within the autistic population than the PNT – autism *is not synonymous* with anxiety, nor does being autistic mean that one will *necessarily* suffer from anxiety. To make it even simpler – again, taking the above into the equation – *anxiety does not stem from being autistic alone*. So we are left with three statements, which all appear to be valid and yet somehow seem contradictory:

1 being autistic means one is at high risk of anxiety;
2 autism and anxiety seem firmly linked;
3 being autistic does not definitively lead to anxiety.

But if autism does not (always) lead to anxiety, then why are some autistic people anxious and others not? You may well already have guessed – it's back to the golden equation, autism + environment = outcome. In this case, if the environment is not suitable in some way for the child, then the outcome is anxiety. It is the combination of being autistic in a non-autism-friendly environment that leads to the anxiety, not being autistic per se, which is why not all autistic people are anxious.

---

[1] This book is about autism, and this chapter is about anxiety. I am very aware that the PNT can also suffer from anxiety to the same degree as the autistic population (though possibly for different reasons) and in no way intend to marginalize or not acknowledge this fact.

In a sense this is both rather depressing and rather encouraging. On the one hand, we know that prevalence rates of anxiety states are so high they are almost seen as the 'norm' for the autistic child; on the other hand, we know that if we get it 'right' then there should be no need for the child to be anxious.

At the time of writing (and I hope this will be outdated information sooner rather than later) there is a far higher prevalence of mental health conditions diagnosed within the autistic population than in the PNT. If we accept that autism is not a psychiatric illness and we accept that there is nothing within the autistic brain that would mean the person (I am including all age ranges here) would be susceptible to being psychiatrically ill, then there must be something else at play here. My belief is that the 'something' in this context is the environment. If the environment is not 'right' then the chances of the child developing anxiety or depression are higher than if she is exposed to an environment that meets her needs. This is the same for *any* child. My rationale is that while this is the same for any child, the reason for higher levels of mental ill health for autistic children is that the environment is so often less friendly to them than to their PNT peers. The optimistic way of looking at this is that if we adapt the environment to better suit the autistic child, then the chances of poor mental health will be considerably reduced.

Never underestimate just how stressful the environment can be for the child – and by environment I include everything from the physical environment through to people talking to the child and everything external to the child that the child experiences. Not only can the child experience trauma from isolated incidents (and these need not be anything obvious to the PNT) but I believe that so-called 'low-level trauma' can be a huge longer-term issue – that is, when a child experiences something problematic (or traumatic) not in isolation but on such a frequent basis that it causes deep long-term ill health issues, often related to anxiety. Consider the following.

School hurts. Not figuratively, literally. I am so sensitive to touch that it hurts when people brush past me. Walking down the corridor is a test of will for me – dare I do it? Do I dare wait and then have all the stress of being late for my next class? That causes its own stress, I don't want to break the rules, nor do I want to stand out in any way. But the corridors here are so crowded – I know it'll hurt, but what choice do I have? Everyone else does it without a problem; I am so useless. But it still hurts and it still takes ages to recover. By which time I've got to do it all over again.

This happens every day I go to school. Five days a week, weeks on end, year after year. Is it any wonder I am an anxious child?

The above could reasonably easily be avoided by having staggered transition times in schools, but until we have a better understanding both of sensory issues and of the impact they have on children this is the sort of thing that could have a major impact on the child's life. Imagine that – the simple act of walking down a corridor being equated to long-term damage to mental health – and yet that could be the reality for an autistic child. Changing the environment, therefore, is essential.

So-called 'low-level trauma' can be experienced in so many different ways by the child; the above is just one simple example. It is essential to have the best communication possible with the child so that she is able to indicate when certain activities or environments are causing a problem, as it may well be that these are so under the radar for the majority of the PNT that they go unnoticed.

I believe that the *feelings* of anxiety and the experience of it are both more intense and experienced for a longer period of time than for the PNT on a day-to-day basis. Speaking with autistic adults has led me to believe that the level of anxiety we are referring to here is that where the person is *consciously aware of his or her own anxiety*; for most people, this does not happen very often. That feeling of 'I know I am stressed' doesn't occur, generally, on a day-to-day basis, but it often does for the autistic child. Not only that, but the feeling can be extremely acute – overwhelming at times and even processed as a physical experience. In addition, the duration of anxiety which is triggered by a specific event can be far longer than the equivalent experience for the PNT. One could identify stages of anxiety thus: 'advance anxiety' (anxiety preceding a specific event), 'event-specific anxiety' (anxiety during the event) and 'post-anxiety' (anxiety release after the event).[2] The following is an example of this from a child's perspective.

I get stressed from the moment I know something is going to happen, however distant it might be in the future. People even tell me, 'Don't worry about that now, it's ages away,' but how am I supposed to forget it when I know it is going to happen? And I don't mean I'm stressed now and then – I'm stressed all the time, because it's on my mind all the time. How can it not be? And what you might think causes me anxiety, just because it's the things that worry you, often doesn't; however, the things that do cause me stress are often overlooked by you because they don't seem to cause you any issue. This is a double blow for me: first, it is difficult for you to identify what I find stressful and, second, it's seemingly rather difficult for you to take my anxiety seriously. Trust me, it's very serious indeed.

So if I know something is going to happen – let's say I have to visit cousin Vinnie's house – then from that point I will start to worry. It will take over huge parts of my mental energy and will probably overwhelm me at times. I will be constantly worrying about it – what should I say, who should I say it to, when should I speak, when shouldn't I, what will we eat, will I have to eat in the vicinity of others, how long will we be there for, who else might be there, how long will the journey be, what do I wear, is it OK for me to leave the room to be on my own, if I do leave the room will that be even worse because everyone will notice . . .? The thoughts go on and on, and when I ask for help I get answers like, 'But you like cousin Vinnie', 'You've been there loads of times before', 'Just be yourself', none of which helps in the slightest. Liking him is absolutely irrelevant as far as I am concerned; it may be true but it doesn't help at all with what is causing me stress. Having been there before might help in other circumstances, but just because things went a certain way last time

---

[2] These suggested terms come from Dr Nick Chown.

does not mean they will be similar this time around, so that makes me even more uncertain and hence more stressed. And being myself certainly won't work when all I will want to do is scream the house down so you don't take me!

The level of anxiety continues. Even after the event, I am anxious. I have to revisit every moment to ascertain what I did and try to figure out whether it was 'correct' or not. This anxiety slowly, so slowly, dissipates over the subsequent weeks.

I hide my anxiety well. You don't seem particularly worried about me. You know I'm stressed about the visit because I've told you. But what you don't realize is the impact on me – the depth of anxiety and the duration. You 'see' my elevated angst on the day itself but have very little idea that the day has actually taken over several weeks of my life. I can't blame you – after all, I have got pretty good at hiding how I really feel. What else am I supposed to do?

So anxiety can be felt acutely, on a continuing basis, and the anxiety can last far longer than it might for the PNT, who, almost as soon as an anxiety-inducing time has finished, will relax.

The above example is one which highlights exactly how it is the environment that can be the part of the issue – in this case visiting cousin Vinnie. No visit equals no anxiety. This does not mean that all autistic children need to avoid any situation that might cause anxiety. What it does mean, though, is that anxiety-inducing situations need to be recognized and understood and systems put in place to alleviate them. In this case, for example, my belief – again – is that environment is of absolute importance. Does everyone know and understand the child's autistic needs? If so, then a huge amount of the anxiety can be taken away: if everyone recognizes that the child will need quiet time to himself and that this needs to be proactively provided and absolutely accepted, then much of the stress could be taken away. If conversations were *started* by the child rather than him having to respond to others, if there was a visit that didn't involve a formal, sit-down meal – these are just some components *in this particular example* that might help.

Of course, it is not at all sensible to make the assumption that one's whole life can be spent with adjustments being made by the rest of the world in order to alleviate one person's anxiety – and it might be very useful indeed to help develop skills to engage with the world in a way that keeps anxiety to a minimum – but it is just as important for the world to understand levels of anxiety and the impact these can have, so that a more measured approach can be taken as to what to expose the child to and when to counterbalance that with autism-friendly, stress-free environments.

How does the child know he's anxious?

A huge problem is that feelings are individual, and therefore how does one know that one is experiencing an environment in a different way in comparison to everyone else? See the section on 'Emotions and autism' in Chapter 6, but also be aware that you may need to be rather proactive in 'finding out' whether a child is stressed. Don't assume he will automatically know himself, or even tell you if he is.

Anxiety and cognition

Not that you need any other reason to lower or eradicate anxiety, but it's worth pointing out that any emotional 'spike' is likely to reduce cognitive functioning. In other words, in this context the higher the anxiety, the lower the ability to think; this is why it's such a bad idea to try and discuss anything (however sensible it might seem to you) with a child whose anxiety is through the roof – wait until the child is calm before attempting to discuss anything. Ending up in a face-to-face 'I won't back down' confrontation will not help anyone and there will be no winners.

Theory of global stability

This is more of a hypothesis than a theory; it is a concept that I believe helps explain, in part, the so-called 'resistance to change' which I am convinced ties in very much with anxiety. At the root of the hypothesis is the simple concept that the more 'globally stable' one is, the more chance one has of being comfortable with areas of life that might be problematic. A simple analogy might be money: if you are a millionaire and you accidently lose a pound you are likely not to be affected very much, if at all; if you are destitute and that one pound is all you possess, then the implications of losing it are extreme. From a 'real' perspective, a pound is simply a pound, but the different levels of (in this case financial) stability between the two examples mean that the loss of a pound leads to little or no change in the life of the financially stable millionaire versus a huge impact in the life of the financially unstable poorer person. Continuing with this analogy, if one were to ask the two individuals: 'What difference to your life would that *change* in financial circumstances mean to you?', I would expect that the millionaire might shrug it off and suggest that she wouldn't really be that bothered, whereas the person for whom a pound is his entire savings might answer very differently. In this sense, one could argue that the latter is *resistant to change* – he is extremely resistant to any changes in his financial circumstances – while the millionaire shows little or no resistance to change whatsoever.

Autistic people are seen as being resistant to change – something I don't agree with. They might be resistant to specific types of changes, but this doesn't mean they are generically averse to change. My hypothesis is that the autistic child is resistant to anything that will upset her *stability*.

So where does stability come from? For most of the PNT, stability – in other words, the day-to-day, average chugging along without major stresses – comes from aspects that are so deep-seated that they don't need to consciously worry about them. For example, most of the PNT rarely need to worry about how to communicate, how to socialize, how to understand what is going on around them, but these are the very aspects of living that might be *unstable* for the autistic child. So while the 'average' PNT goes about life in a pretty stable state – and, therefore, doesn't need to worry about minor changes – the autistic child may be in a state of chaos much of the time. If she cannot communicate effectively, if she does not socialize in the same way as the majority, if she does not understand the world around her because the unwritten rules are PNT-based, not autism-friendly, then her daily life's stability is likely to depend very strongly on a very few elements. My understanding is that *those* elements are either things that remain the same every day (or seem to) and/or things that are totally in the control of the autistic child. These, in the great scheme of things, are usually very few and far between.

What this means is that, over a period of, for example, a day, there is very little that the child can actually 'rely on' to provide a sense of stability. What this also means is that the things that do provide stability – much like the poor person's last pound – become incredibly important. If *those* things were to change – well, that's when acute levels of distress can be seen, even though to the external observer the change appears to be both trivial and minor. Here is an example.

> My day is chaotic. It often starts with yet another different instruction from Dad; everything looks different, feels different, my school uniform smells different, even Mum's voice is different in the morning compared to what it sounded like last night. Each school day will be different. I don't really understand how to get on with my classmates – there is so little I can rely on. Still, at least the route to school and back is nice and predictable. Same route each day – it gives me at least some stability throughout the day that I can rely on, even though it's just 20 minutes each way. That's 40 minutes of relax time, which just about counterbalances all that goes on in between.

For this child, then, imagine what happens when there is a road diversion. All of a sudden, the only thing he could rely on for stability for that period of time is taken away from him. His reaction – perfectly understandable under the circumstances – might be extreme. After all, how would most people react if their stability was massively interrupted and ripped away from them? But society might not see that; instead, people might simply suggest he's 'resistant to change' because he likes his routine to school. What they don't understand is that the only thing the child can rely on for that day has been taken away from him.

Of course, there are all sorts of other reasons why a child might like a routine, but for many children the routines are there because their levels of global stability are so low that they *need* predictability and routine in order to feel even a little bit stable. What the child 'sees' as stable is very individual (although I did choose the route to school deliberately as it's so common!). The point is, if a child demonstrates this 'resistance to change' and it can be identified that the reason behind this is a lack of global stability, then the response may need to be somewhat considered. Often the reaction is, 'Well, the world is not a perfect place so he needs to understand we can't go the same way to school every day,' but this, to me, is missing the point entirely. The child doesn't want or need to go to school via the same route every day in order to feel safe – he needs to feel safe so that he *doesn't* need to go to school via the same route every day. We can only manage that by understanding what is chaotic in the child's life and addressing that.

'She needs to learn'

This is such a common reaction to anxiety that I feel it warrants a section in its own right. It is so often that a reaction to anxiety is a far too simplistic declaration that the child simply has to learn that this is the way of the world, and needs to get used to it, learn to cope with it, adapt to it. I am not suggesting that autistic children can't learn, nor that they don't have to, in some ways – everyone does, to a degree. However, it is essential in supporting the autistic child to understand that he or she will not become 'less autistic' by default simply through being exposed to a stressful situation over and over again until it all of a sudden becomes acceptable. Yes, children *do* need to learn – of course they do. But the way in which they are supported to do so is crucial, not just in terms of success but in terms of reducing risk of damage to the autistic child's mental well-being.

Rather than identifying an aspect of life which could be seen as something the child relies on and then 'teaching' alternatives, a far more effective strategy might be to recognize that the *reason* the route to school is so important is that the child finds the school bit in between so chaotic. Ascertaining what particular aspects of school life are chaotic and addressing them successfully might be a more difficult way forward than 'teaching' an alternative route to school, but in the long run it is a far more effective support for the child. Rather than 'making the child cope', one is, instead, addressing the underlying cause of stress. If this is done well then – without any other 'intervention' – the need for the route to school to stay the same will reduce naturally, as the child no longer 'needs' it for his stability.

Please note: sometimes a supportive environment exposing the child to new or stressful activities in a manner that allows him, in his own time, to get used to it and develop confidence can be an excellent way forward in nurturing him; my point above is that if there is a very specific reason behind the anxiety, then the anxiety is unlikely to diminish simply by exposure to it.

Masking

Also known as copying, or what I refer to as echopraxia, masking is the deliberate action of the autistic person to copy the PNT in daily life. It can be an extraordinarily tiring thing to do: constantly working out how to act based on one's experience of 'people-watching' can be an exhausting way of engaging with the world. For some people, masking can be a brilliant way of 'getting along' without standing apart as the odd one out, but is this always necessarily a good thing?

Why do I mask?

- I mask to try and fit in.
- I mask because if I don't I will get sectioned.
- I mask because otherwise children laugh at me.
- I mask because otherwise my behaviour will be seen as an indication of a mental disorder.
- I mask because how else am I supposed to know how to behave?
- I mask because I hate the spotlight.
- I mask because society has shamed me into doing so.
- I mask because *you* tell me I need to behave differently from what is natural to me.

Example of masking

> I'm in the classroom again. Another day, another problem. Every class is different – different teacher, different kids, different rules, different ways of listening, different ways of talking. It's literally so different that I have no clue what is expected of me. I hate standing out, but I know I will unless I 'conform' – and yet I don't know how to conform as I don't understand all the unwritten rules. What I do know is that Jane over there never gets picked up by the teacher for doing anything wrong; she ticks along quite nicely without a care in the world. I copy her in as much detail as I possibly can. By doing so, I also escape the teacher's attention – and I can finally relax.

In the short term, masking can be a great way of being. It solves all sorts of problems. However, longer term this may not be a positive way of 'coping' with the world; the longer one masks, the less time one spends being oneself and the greater the risk of losing a sense of self and who one actually is. Everyone masks to a certain degree, but autistic people may do so way beyond what the PNT would ordinarily ever do, and do so far more deliberately and with the need for expenditure of a huge amount of intellectual and emotional energy. This latter cannot be overestimated.

While some children appear to use masking effectively, it is also well worth considering the fact that autistic children need time to be themselves. Again, everyone will declare at times that 'they need time to be themselves' – particularly (perhaps ironically) after a time of intense social interaction, when one can hear the PNT declare, 'I can't wait to get home for some alone time' – and yet how much time do we proactively afford our autistic children to be themselves, and to *enjoy* being themselves, without judgement?

Meltdowns

Sometimes children will suffer from such levels of anxiety or sensory overload that they may lose control of their own behaviour and a meltdown might occur. Please note: *a meltdown is categorically not a tantrum*. The latter implies a level of control or manipulation or deliberate use of behaviour; a meltdown is not the same thing at all, irrespective of how it might be displayed. A meltdown is a reaction to extreme levels of stress and should be absolutely acknowledged as such. If a child is in meltdown mode then it is likely to be an indication that something is very wrong indeed. Trying to 'punish' a meltdown or similar is not only highly unlikely to 'work' but may be utterly unfair on the autistic child, who is likely to feel utterly drained following a meltdown, let alone completely negative towards herself for something she has no control over anyway.

If a child is having a meltdown then she will probably need time to herself – safely – to recover. I deliberately won't write 'time to calm down' as again this suggests some level of anger or deliberate behaviour. A meltdown indicates loss of control resulting from absolute overload; so many PNT cannot understand this, for the simple fact that they have never experienced, even in all their years, such levels of distress that they have entered meltdown mode. Recovery may take some while, and the child needs absolute reassurance that the meltdown is in no way a fault of hers. Understanding how to avoid meltdowns by recognizing that they stem from stress is a huge step towards a happy autistic child!

What is a meltdown?

There are so many ways in which a meltdown might manifest; some you will be aware of in no uncertain terms but others may be out of sight. This does not mean that they should be out of mind! It is tempting to assume that the more 'dramatic' the meltdown (self-injury, screaming and so on – the sorts of things that are extremely tough to witness), the more distressed the child. This may not be the case. The withdrawal, the loss of speech, the sudden decrease in motivation – these may also indicate meltdown-type experiences. As noted, meltdowns are the direct result of extreme distress. The way in which children react will differ from one to the next, but irrespective of the way in which a meltdown is displayed (or not), each instance must be taken seriously.

Other causes of anxiety

Communication

Children will range from being non-verbal to verbose. This does not mean one child has more or less effective communication than another, nor will it indicate levels of anxiety related to it. In fact, a verbal child may have more anxiety related to speech, as there will be higher expectations for her to use it, despite the fact that PNT language can be highly baffling and, therefore, anxiety-inducing!

> *Teacher*: Class, time to finish.
> *Teacher*: Jane, I've told you to finish!
> *Jane*: No you didn't, my name isn't 'class'.
> *Teacher*: Don't be so cheeky, you'll get into trouble!

Jane ends the school day wondering, yet again, why being accurate with language has got her into trouble.

This is just such a simple example of how a misunderstanding might take place; no one is at fault, and yet it is usually the autistic child who ends up with the blame.

Accurate processing of language – or, according to a negative pathology, 'literal interpretation of language' (which in itself, ironically, is somewhat linguistically dubious – if one is literal can one also be interpreting?) – can cause all sorts of problems when the main protagonists are those who say things that are either clearly not linguistically accurate, or are ambiguous or, simply, are not true. Telling a child that you'll do it 'in a minute' may result in a distrust in your ability to tell the time. You reassuring your wife that she has not put on any weight may result in your child disbelieving anything else you might say. You changing your mind after laying down a rule and subsequently changing it might mean the child never again 'believes' in a rule.

These examples may be somewhat extreme, but the essence is there. Imagine a world in which a child knows the following three facts.

1 I know people say things that turn out to be true.
2 I know people say things that turn out to be false.
3 I have no idea how to ascertain whether or not a person is trustworthy in what he or she says.

This puts the child in a horribly compromising situation. Imagine not knowing whether or not you can genuinely trust what a person says, as you know she sometimes says things that are true but equally sometimes says things that are false. It can be massively anxiety-inducing.

It is useful from as early an age as possible to accept that there will be language differences between your child and others, and that while it may cause issues, there are ways to reduce those differences. Acknowledging that PNT language is a minefield and often inaccurate is a great starting point: it is extremely frustrating for the autistic child to hear comments such as 'Well, you must know what I mean' or similar – if he did, there wouldn't be any issue! Taking responsibility for the fact that you may say something that turns out to be inaccurate is a good way to develop trust; the opposite will happen if you insist that you are right all the time when, from an autism perspective, you may not be.

Having a small number of trusted confidantes (often parents) can be an absolute joy: people who will listen and explore the issues from an 'autistically honest' perspective. Allies like this are something that many autistic people may not have access to, but they are invaluable when it comes to reducing anxiety.

Incidentally, lying can be a baffling concept to many autistic children (and adults), including the 'white lie'. Imagine what a strange world it is, taking the below example, from an autism perspective.

So weird. Mum asked Dad if he thought she had put on weight. Why she asked him in the first place, I have no idea. I mean, I see her weighing herself pretty much obsessively, and the bathroom scales live next to a pretty big mirror so surely she must have a bit of a clue. Not only that, but she had to buy new clothes since she stopped that diet of hers, and seeing as they are a size bigger than last year – well, enough said. Anyway, even more bizarre than her asking Dad was his response: he said, 'No, dear, of course not.' I mean, what? Not only such a whopper of a lie, but what did he mean, 'Of course not'? I would have thought the opposite should have been the honest answer, as in, 'Of course you have – what do you expect after having given up your diet?' or something similar. Still, each to their own, I suppose. What I just don't get, after why she asked in the first place, then why he clearly lied, is that they both seem quite happy with each other, when lying is supposed to be such a no-go area for a happy marriage! I get told to tell the truth all the time, yet when others lie it's apparently OK!

This example demonstrates just how bewildering the PNT life can be to the autistic child, which can, in turn, lead to anxiety. In this case, how is the child supposed to know when it is or isn't OK to lie?

As noted, having a person as the 'go-to' individual 'allows' the child to essentially listen to what others have to say and then ask for it to be translated by a trusted person. This kind of 'interpreter' can work in so many different levels for the child – not just language, but social situations as well. It might be that you think the child needs to be 'independent', but almost everyone has a support system around them, even as adults. Why can't the autistic child have one too?

Other aspects to consider to reduce anxiety

These include the following.

- Understanding the environment – rules and regulations. Does the child know what to expect and how to deal with it in any given environment?
- Understanding what is expected of me. Does the child understand the expectations on him?
- Being able to comfortably process the sensory environment. Is the sensory environment appropriate or does it have appropriate escape areas that are known to the child?
- Whether any expectations the child has prior to an event are fulfilled or not.
- Knowing how to engage with my environment and having an escape clause wherever possible. Does the child have an 'out' at all times to allow anxiety to be kept at a minimum?

- Being effective with contingency plans so the unexpected becomes the expected. Are there clear contingency plans so that if things change there are still identified plans that can be adhered to?

6

Happy autistic children

Rationale

I hate to mention it, but very often – far too often – autistic children are not as happy as their PNT counterparts. The previous chapter has identified many of the reasons why the child may be anxious; this chapter aims to take a broader perspective in terms of how society might adapt and change in order to create a culture of happiness within the autistic population. I fully believe that children will be impacted by the general attitude towards them of those around them, starting off with those closest to them and all the way through to media and exposure in wider society. So, clearly, there is a long way to go, but in identifying at least some of the aspects related to autism, we as a society can start to change, we can attempt to ensure that children have a brighter future. This is just one example – it's actually a tweet I sent out on social media.

> Little plea to all autism resources, schools, etc. PLEASE remove all references to 'disorder' in your literature, particularly posters that can be seen in class. Autistic kids really don't need to be reading that they are disordered every day they attend school!

Taking a step back and thinking about this, even just for a few seconds, makes me realize just how influential – often without realizing it – practice can be on the very population we are trying to support. The tweet arose after I had visited many schools, all of which were trying to best support their autistic pupils and all of which 'raised awareness' in various ways, including having posters up about autism. Every single one of them referred to autism as a disorder. Just imagine what it must be like to be exposed to that kind of negativity – however well-meaning – on pretty much a daily basis. Being given the message, however unintentionally, that you, as an autistic child in this school, are a *disordered* person is not particularly pleasant, I would imagine, let alone the far more long-term implications of what this might mean to a child's self-esteem and mental health. Changing the way in which we adopt language does make a difference!

This chapter aims to identify certain broad notions and concepts that need to change in order for us to nurture whole generations of happy autistic children. Some of them need society's recognition while some of them can be applied on an individual basis, day to day. Some may appear (or even are) rather optimistic, but that doesn't invalidate them!

Paradigm shift in the concept and understanding of autism

Following on from the above, I believe it is about time that the world as a whole had a paradigm shift in its understanding of autism. How this might come about I am less sure, I have to admit! But it would be fantastic if autism could be reframed to sit outside of medicalized volumes that pathologize and make negative what could otherwise be understood as a cognitive difference instead of a deficit state. How this might come about, as I stated, I am not yet sure, but consider the fact that homosexuality was medicalized as a psychiatric condition within recent times. This has now drastically changed, and one might conclude that perhaps autism could or should be going the same way – that is, that it should no longer be pathologized as some kind of mental illness that needs curing.

Incidentally, just as an example of how medicalized and pathologized autism currently is, within the UK we have the Equality Act (2010), and other countries have similar legislation (though not all). Essentially, one *should not* be discriminated against as a result of:

- age
- disability
- gender reassignment
- marriage and civil partnership
- pregnancy and maternity

- race
- religion or belief
- sex
- sexual orientation.

This is great, but what is less impressive is the requirement of 'proof'. As far as I know, one does not have to have a 'diagnosis' of being gay to warrant protection from this legislation. Nor a diagnosis of being a woman. Nor of being from an ethnic minority, and so on. One does, however, in some circumstances need a medical corroboration of being autistic before one can be protected. Is this fair? Is it, in fact, 'equal'? I absolutely recognize that there are all sorts of arguments about the need for a 'diagnosis', but I am also of the belief that the requirement for one, without the (legal) fallback position of simply 'knowing' one is autistic (self-diagnosed) might well put many autistic people at a huge disadvantage and left unprotected by the very legislation that is supposed to ensure that they are not discriminated against.

   In relation to autism, though, what we need as a society is a pretty much complete transformation within society as to how autism is viewed, from a negative, medical model or misguided savant-type population to a recognition that, actually, being autistic only tells us that a person is autistic – in the same way that, without knowing a person, being informed that she is black, he is gay, she is 33 years old, he is Catholic tells you nothing other than exactly that! Until society absolutely accepts that the identity of autism should not be associated with 'lesser' in any automatic way, then children will be likely to be at the sharp end of the metaphorical stick.

Stop comparing to the PNT – or other autistic children

This section is an adaptation from a blog post I wrote and follows on very much from the point above.

Why do autistics need to be compared to the PNT?

This has been worrying me a lot recently. The whole notions of diagnosis (or, of course, identification) through to reasonable adjustments, the concept of disability, equality, fairness – to me a lot of the issues stem from what I see as a fundamental and critical flaw in how autistic people are commonly compared to the PNT, as opposed to simply being understood within their own context. One only needs to scan through definitions and descriptors of autism to ascertain just how much judgement of the autistic person there is in relation to the PNT. Impairment in social skills? Read as impairment in PNT social skills. Impairment in theory of mind? Read impairment in PNT theory of mind. The list could go on . . . and on. The point is that these judgements mostly seem to be a direct comparative analysis of so-called skill sets against a demographic majority – which holds absolutely no logic whatsoever. It's akin to deciding that the lone dog in a room full of cats should be described as having impairments in purring, meowing and looking aloof (slight sarcasm warning for that last sentence, by the way). I am not for one moment suggesting that autistic kids are a different species from the PNT, but should their identity essentially stem from a comparative analysis of skills profiles compared to their non-autistic counterparts? I am not in the least bit convinced that this should be the case. However, I have covered much of this earlier in the book. What I wanted to consider here is how the autistic child is also compared – not neurologically in this instance but in 'performance' – not against what I might consider to be an appropriate set of criteria but against a 'standardized' set of criteria that may be completely inappropriate to that child's goals.

Anyway, I shall get to the point that has been worrying me recently. It's this: that the autistic person's success or otherwise is based on *PNT perception and status*, as opposed to autistic potential. This scares me beyond belief, as it might mean that autistic children and adults are at a massive disadvantage just because they are able to 'perform' at a similar level to their PNT peers. If this is the case, then society is getting things very wrong indeed. Take the following examples:

- a child in a mainstream school, causing no fuss, passing her coursework and exams with average marks;
- an employee with no remarkable productivity but with no obvious negative issues either;
- a university student, on for a below-average second-class degree.

One might argue that if all three of the above were autistic, it is unlikely that they would 'qualify' for any additional support, reasonable adjustment, application of equality laws and so on – after all, what's the problem? Well, for me, the problem is that those individuals are being judged or assessed against a 'norm' *and not against their own potential*. If being autistic is holding them back because of a lack of adjustment, then they are at a grave disadvantage. If, with reasonable adjustment, those three could be the straight 'A' child in school, the most productive employee, the first-class honours student, then are we not being discriminatory by failing to recognize this and failing to do something about it?

The same applies to being identified as autistic in the first place. One tends to need to be perceived as disabled in the first instance to 'qualify' for a diagnosis: 'persistent difficulties . . . impairments . . .' and so on – but compared to what? Or, more importantly, compared to whom? What if we radically changed our perception and instead asked the question: how much less disadvantaged might an individual be if we took autism into account, even if there appears to be no issue on the surface? You might have a child who does not outwardly demonstrate a persistent difficulty in effective communication, but compared to her potential she may be operating at a considerably lower level because autism has not been identified or taken into account. Surely what this means is that the way we (society in general) understand and perceive autism should be vastly different compared to current thinking. One should not have to demonstrate disability, difficulty or impairment to qualify either for a diagnosis or for reasonable support to reach your child's own potential, not what is deemed appropriate or acceptable for the PNT.

What I believe is required is a level of expertise in terms of (1) what is important and (2) what is potential – and neither of these should be based on PNT norms.

What is important simply has to take the autistic child into account. It may be hugely important for the child to have 'downtime' in order to balance out the considerable chaos of the outside world. We live in a society whereby there are certain notions that seem to be based on very little in terms of validity – notions such as 'he shouldn't spend so much time alone', 'she needs a lot of friends' or 'being independent is a useful goal to aim for'. These, I believe, are based on PNT philosophy and are aimed at achieving well-being – for example, PNTs are usually extremely socially driven – so spending time with others and having friends might be an indication of a rewarding existence. The problem – and it's a huge problem – stems from the erroneous assumption that children need to demonstrate these indicators for their well-being to be achieved. In other words, spending time with others and having friends will lead to a contented child. This *may* not be the case at all for the autistic child, whose parameters are completely different and who cannot (or, rather, should not) be 'judged' by the same indicators. In fact, the child might strive to have time alone, and may be absolutely at ease and relaxed while this is the case; this doesn't mean he doesn't enjoy friends or having company, but the way in which he does so may differ considerably from the PNT, and this should be respected and taken into account at all times. Of course, some autistic children will love time with others and this may then become an indicator of their well-being, but the concept as a whole cannot be applied successfully to all children.

Potential is an area that might be rather difficult to judge. My view is that potential should always be assumed to be infinite, otherwise subconscious barriers could be put in place in terms of expectation and the child might then never go beyond those barriers. But having faith that your child's abilities are limitless should not mean that expectations are equally high – there is a fine balance between allowing your child to develop (at a pace that suits her) and being disappointed if expectations are unrealistic. So many parents get surprised by their amazing children later on in life; I genuinely believe that the whole way of autistic learning (in all aspects of learning, not just education) differs so greatly from the PNT, and reflected in this is the way in which those kids develop. Using a PNT standard against how a child reaches certain milestones, develops and works her way through life in general can be massively unfair to that child. So long as you are confident that your child is going in the right direction then it is perfectly acceptable not to compare her against what other PNT kids are up to. Happiness is far more important than pretty much anything else.

Understanding self and others

As noted in Chapter 2, an understanding of self is critical for the autistic child. Not knowing one is autistic and thus making problematic assumptions about yourself can lead to so many issues around sense of self and self-esteem. Here is an imaginary story that I hope explains, in part at least, what some of the issues might be.

Deep underground there lived a society of beings that dwelt within the rocks and burrows and caves that their forebears had spent hundreds of years creating; no one knew how the beings came to live so far within the ground, and no one ever asked – it was accepted as 'just the way it is and always has been', for this was the way of the gloobs, as they were known. Gloobs were fairly simple creatures; they found nourishment in the water that trickled down through the roof of their caves and they spent their time huddled together for warmth and company, whiling the time away by chatting about who had the biggest cave, who had the best water supply, who liked whom the most, what changes in temperature there had been that day (the answer was always the same as the temperature never changed) and other such innocuous chatter that they loved so much. None of the gloobs ever really thought about why they were there, where they had come from and what the future held for them. They were perfectly content huddling, chatting and drinking. They absolutely loved their social lives and, most of all, they loved to gossip and joke with one another.

However, there was one gloob who just didn't seem to fit in. From an early age she just didn't seem to want to do the same things as other gloobs: she didn't like huddling as she said it made her skin ache; she didn't talk much at all and, when she did, she showed a rather worrying (to others) inquisitiveness that disturbed the other gloobs – for example, she wanted to know where the water came from and what might be above the dwellings. She seemed far more interested in examining her surroundings than chatting to her peers. She preferred not to joke and had a reputation for seriousness, which was not altogether fair as she had a rather fun sense of humour, but she tended to keep herself to herself so none of the other gloobs knew about it. Her name was Samuit – or Sammy, as she liked to be known.

At first, Sammy had a good life. The other gloobs didn't really pay her much attention and were far too busy chatting with one another to notice this little gloob, especially as she spent so much time in the corners of the caves or staring up at the ceilings, tracing water trickles with her eyes. But as time went on and little Sammy started to turn into a young lady gloob, the differences in her nature became more and more apparent. She was frequently asked why she didn't behave in the same way as everyone else and was even told off for spending so much time on her own, staring at the water. Sammy was very, very upset by this. She didn't see what the problem was – she wasn't, after all, doing anyone any harm. In fact, she was beginning to notice that the water trickles were changing in their behaviour and she had all sorts of queries and thoughts and suppositions as to why this might be, all of which were far more interesting than having to listen to the other gloobs boasting about the size of their caves. She didn't know why she should be told off and it made her very miserable. She tried talking to her fellow gloobs about the water, but no one seemed interested and some even teased her about her 'water obsession'.

Eventually, young Sammy was told by the Elders that she needed to stop worrying about the water and must come along to the group huddle and chat with everyone else about who had the biggest cave. Sammy tried. She tried so, *so* hard, but she couldn't bear the feeling of the huddle. She didn't need it for warmth as she was never cold anyway and she simply couldn't follow the conversations at all; they all seemed to be pointless nonsense to her, so when others told her it was her turn, she froze and couldn't speak. While no one said anything to her about this, it made her feel terrible. 'Why can't I be like them?' she thought. And Sammy became very sad indeed. In fact, she was so sad, she decided that she had to leave the community.

Sammy travelled far and wide, along forgotten pathways and burrows. Whenever there was a choice, she would take the path that led upwards, as she was convinced there were answers to her questions that she could seek. She constantly worried about the water trickles and why they were diminishing. She loved her community, even though she didn't always understand it, and while none of them seemed worried, she was. She was lonely, it's true, and she always had the nagging thoughts about why she couldn't fit in, but her focus was 'onwards and upwards': she felt she had a purpose and she wanted answers.

A year later, long after the furore of Sammy leaving the gloob community had died down, the gloobs were in a bad way. The water had near enough stopped trickling through their ceilings and their conversations during huddle time frequently turned to Sammy and how she had been the first to notice. They felt very sorry that they had not listened to her and they said to each other that they had been too harsh to dismiss her behaviour as odd when, in fact, it seemed as though she had had something important to say. How they missed Sammy and wished they had been kinder and more accepting – after all, she might have the answer to their problem.

And she did.

Sammy returned, with tales of the amazing times she had had, all the adventures she had been on, but most importantly, with news as to where all the water had gone. She knew that the gloobs were stuck in their ways and didn't like to be exposed too much, too quickly to anyone different from them, so she figured out a way to protect them from the wider world while ensuring that they had enough water. It was Sammy who made the negotiations with the Upper World, as it became known; it was Sammy who acted as the bridge between the gloobs and the big wide world; and it was Sammy who saved the gloobs from a very unpleasant future.

Sammy lived a long and happy life. On her travels she had realized that, while she was just as much a gloob as the rest of them, the fact that she thought and experienced the world in a different way didn't make her bad, just different. And it was because of those differences that she was able to have such an impact on her little community. Being away from the community had allowed Sammy to reflect on herself and realize that being a bit different didn't make her in the least bit bad; and Sammy being away also made the community realize that they missed her interesting ways of looking at things that were different from their own perspective. No longer did the other gloobs tease her – quite the opposite! While the gloobs were often so stuck in their ways, Sammy had taught them a valuable lesson about how all communities need gloobs who think and act just a bit differently from everyone else.

What is worrying is that there are very few resources to support autistic children in having that understanding of self that might assist in a more positive feeling about who one is. Certainly, there are campaigns within the wider community about 'autism awareness' and suchlike, though it is not clear just how effective these are in helping the world understand *your* child; yet where are the resources to teach autistic children about themselves – and, just as important, where are the resources to teach autistic children about the PNT?

Imagine a world where you are the odd one out. Would it be helpful to be taught why all the others behave in the way they do? To have explanations as what those differences are and how they manifest? How you could make sense of them? I suspect it would be at the very least a huge relief to have a better understanding of the people around you, if not a life-saver! And yet we don't habitually teach children the 'way of the PNT' in a formal and useful way.

In order to develop a healthy, happy, autistic community we need to teach fundamental aspects of life which could include:

- what it means to you – individually – to be autistic;
- why you should not compare yourself against your PNT peers;
- why you should not compare yourself against your autistic peers either.

The latter is important. Once a child understands that she is autistic and has been given the go-ahead to stop comparing herself with a set of criteria that is not appropriate, the temptation might be to seek alternative criteria against which to judge self – and that temptation might stem from looking to the rest of the autistic population. Sometimes this can be an extremely affirming process: meeting like-minded people, reading their stories, sharing experiences – these can all be extremely beneficial. The problem arises, though, when a child has recognized her identity but then comes across information that makes her doubt it all over again; those worries that 'Well, she's autistic and she can do that, but I'm rubbish at it' can become problematic in and of themselves and leave the child in a state of unknowing all over again. So, while it can be so wonderful for autistic children to engage with the rest of the autistic population, they need to do so with a full understanding that there will be differences even within that population as well as with the wider PNT.

What does understanding of self entail?

One of the most important things for any child is to understand self. This *must* be developed at an individual level as self is, by definition, individual! Children need to understand the appropriate set of criteria against which to judge the self in order to be happy. If they continually judge themselves against a PNT set of criteria, they are very likely to 'fail', leading them to think that they are not particularly successful (or, worse, it can have a hugely negative impact on self-worth and self-esteem and even lead to poor mental well-being). I think that a (relatively) simple way of existing on a day-to-day basis is to constantly and proactively ask the self questions – so long as there is continuing support for the child in how to answer them, and so long as every question takes the child's own strengths and weaknesses into account. The questions that could be asked of the self around any decision could be ones such as the following.

- What is the short-term and long-term impact of the decision on me?
- What is the short-term and long-term impact of the decision on others?
- Am I making the decision taking into account the moral and ethical parameters that I subscribe to?

If the child has been enabled to develop a set of parameters that she is satisfied and comfortable with, even if a decision 'goes wrong', at least she knows that she has done everything in her power to get it 'right'. Every decision can be a learning curve, and those parameters or boundaries can adapt over time as development, understanding, motivation (and so on) change – the point being that, should things in life go wrong (as they often do), if the child has a system he trusts and adheres to, then he doesn't need to constantly blame himself, or ruminate for hours on end as to why something went wrong.

This 'system' may not be for everyone, and it is not easy to implement! But it can be an absolute lifeline for children for whom how to monitor self and make decisions might otherwise be extremely problematic.

Concept to question: friends are a necessity

As alluded to several times already, the 'value judgements' that are so instilled into us from a very early age need to be questioned. One of these judgements is that to be healthy (emotionally, socially, mentally) one needs friends – there is almost an unspoken agreement, in fact, that there is a correlation between the number of friends one has and the level of positive feeling one might expect. While this might be the case for many of the PNT (and I'm not even that convinced it is anyway), we absolutely cannot make the assumption that the same will apply to autistic children. Here are some categorical facts that will apply to some autistic children (of course, the list is not exhaustive).

- Some children simply do not want friends.
- Some children only want one friend.
- Some children want 'friends', but their view of what makes a friend may differ considerably from that of a more general consensus.
- Some children have no friends but are desperately lonely.
- Some children have no friends and try hard to get them, with little or no success.
- Some children have friends and are very happy with what they have.

What might apply to your child may well change over time as well – just to complicate things!

Not wanting friends

One of the things that some parents might find difficult to accept is that, actually, their child is perfectly OK with being on his own or mingling with family members, but without a friend to speak of. The important phrase here is 'perfectly happy' – if a child is perfectly happy then why feel the need to change anything? Just because his circumstance might not make others happy, if he is content then there is no discernible problem!

Wanting one friend

Lots of children find that one friend at a time is exactly what is required to meet their needs. In fact, some autistic logic might state that any more than one friend is a 'waste' – why spend energy on more than one person at a time? Others might feel that a single friend keeps things nice and simple, and they may have a very valid point. After all, the change in social dynamics moving from a couple to a triumvirate can be considerable!

However, having one friend, while it may suit the child magnificently, may not always be what is best for the friend. Sometimes, as a parent, one needs to be supportive in terms of guiding the child as to how 'full on' or otherwise one needs to be in order to keep a friendship going. This isn't to say that there is a right or wrong way to be a friend, but the autistic way of being a friend may differ considerably from the PNT expectation, in which case, sometimes, difficulties may arise. So a child may appear to be either rather overwhelming or overbearing (wanting lots of time and attention from her friend) or appear to almost be the opposite, as if she is indifferent, and may only make contact when it suits her. Of course, there is plenty of autistic logic behind both ways of being, but the PNT friend may not quite see it like that.

Wanting 'alternative' friends

Some children have quite fixed ideas as to what they want out of a friend – which makes perfect sense, and yet society may not deem this OK, for whatever reason. So, some children may see a person as their 'videogaming friend' and engage in one particular interest with that person, but have several other friends who meet other needs. I think this is somewhat similar to how PNT adults behave, which just shows how advanced in development some autistic children actually are! In a similar vein, autistic children may disregard illogical (to them) aspects of the friend, such as age. To them, it is a specific defining factor that makes the person a friend, and this may have nothing to do with age.

There is a strong argument to suggest that any peer should be identified on a person-to-person basis, *not* within a group population. To try and identify an entire group who are likely to be compatible with the autistic child is hugely problematic. It may well be that a peer who is eminently suitable for one aspect of life (say, social activity) might be entirely negative in another (say, academic study). A 'starter' list of aspects that might need to be taken into account when trying to identify peers includes compatibility in:

- emotional understanding;
- social needs;
- sense of humour;
- academic ability (and this can then be broken down by subject, so one person may be compatible in maths, but the child may need an alternative academic peer in languages);
- motivation or sharing of an interest;
- communicative method or understanding;
- play activity;
- sensory processing;
- attention span.

Some autistic children thoroughly enjoy the company of the older generation, with whom they may engage extremely well; some (or the same child) may enjoy time with a much younger generation. The point is, many autistic children will – in an autistically logical way – not view age as a particularly important aspect when engaging with others; in fact, some may be as logical as to suggest that age has literally got nothing whatsoever to do with whether or not a person is the right one to connect with. From an autism perspective this seems eminently sensible – and, in fact, it often is – but, of course, one needs to take safety issues into account at all times.

No friends, but lonely

This is a dangerous state to be in. Do not make the mistake of assuming that because a child seeks solitude then it automatically means she wants it. It might be that she is doing so not because she doesn't want friends, but for a bunch of other reasons – usually negative. Examples might include:

- no idea how to go about finding or making or keeping friends;
- tried before (once) and it didn't work so assume it's never going to work;
- too terrifying;
- not sure who is eligible;
- too much conflicting advice;
- looks far too complicated.

If your child needs support to find, make or maintain a friend rather than being content on his own, then a very different approach will be required.

No friends, but trying to get them

Your child does want friends but is not being successful. There is much literature out there that might help, and this area could be a book in its own right – but identifying compatibility for different areas of life could be incredibly useful, rather than trying to find the one person who will meet all your child's needs in one go. It might be that you try to find someone who will be interested in the same activity as your child, in which case the focus could be on the activity rather than the social side of things (which takes a lot of pressure off the social side of things). Then you may search for a compatible person with whom to do an alternative activity, and so on. For instance, the chess club might be good for one thing, while an online 'friend' for gaming might meet a need for another.

Just a quick note on virtual relationships: online engagement is a valid form of social interaction. Assuming that safeguards are in place, just because a child is 'alone' in his bedroom does not mean that he is isolated and 'cut off' from the world. If he is online with 'friends' – even if he's never met them – then it is likely to be a very healthy and positive experience, particularly if the alternative is sitting at home in his bedroom genuinely alone. Just because a relationship is 'alternative' does not invalidate it in the slightest.

Another note: there appears to be a general consensus that 'screen time is bad'. This is a massive oversimplification. Of course, it may be bad in some circumstances, but in others it may be wholly positive. I hope the theme of this book is clear: never make assumptions about your child based on concepts devised by the PNT and aimed at the PNT population!

Friends and happy

Great – but make sure your child has support in discussing how relationships are going, as sometimes being able to identify and predict possible pitfalls can help avoid them occurring!

Finally for this section on friends: people might ask, 'Who is best as a friend, another autistic child or not?' Of course, there is no right or wrong answer. It might be that having an autistic friend could be hugely beneficial, especially if they share similar experiences that will allow a certain level of familiarity and reduce the feeling of thinking one is very much on one's own in the world, while having a good PNT friend could act as a fantastic conduit between the autistic child and a wider social experience – the most important component, quite simply, is the happiness of the child.

Concept to question: assessments are valid for all neurotypes

We 'assess' kids frequently, in all sorts of ways, from weighing and measuring as an infant, through developmental milestones, to exams at university and interview panels for jobs. This is fine; in many ways assessments can be helpful, valid ways of understanding useful information. However, a word of warning: if an assessment (in its loosest definition) has been developed by the PNT for the PNT (which means most assessments) then the outcomes of those assessments when applied to the autistic child may not be as valid as they are for the PNT. This will not benefit the happiness of the autistic child if he is 'failing' assessments constantly, not because he is defective in any way but because of the way in which the assessment has taken place. A perhaps obvious example of this might be a simple question such as the following on a worksheet in a classroom.

Can you draw a circle around all the numbers you can see in the picture?

Of course, the answer is simply 'yes' or 'no', but most PNT children would understand the terribly unclear language and 'interpret' it for what it actually means (an instruction rather than a question). With a 'yes', though, the autistic child may get a rather negative response, despite the very honest and accurate answer. In this sense the child may 'fail' the assessment, despite demonstrating possibly superior language skills to his teacher!

I would argue that every single 'assessment', from speech and language assessments to developmental milestones to PhD vivas, needs to be understood, adapted and contextualized (or completely rewritten or developed) to take any specific autistic person into account. After all, we already know that autistic children develop faster in some areas and slower in others, that language development differs considerably and that any 'traditional' viva structure might require reasonable adjustments in order not to discriminate against the autistic student – so, surely, any general assessment instrument should require careful consideration prior to validating it for the autistic population.

Many tests and exams seem to me to ascertain, at least to some degree, the ability of the child to respond *to that test or exam* – and not, as the test or exam might purport, the skill level of the child in that subject area. One prime example is the autistic child taking a maths exam. He answered *every single question* correctly – and yet 'scored' relatively low marks. The reason for this was that the exam was marked in a certain way, including the allocation of marks for 'showing the working out'. When questioned, the child very (autistically) logically noted that he must be able to work out the answers – otherwise how else would he have got them correct? – so demonstrating this in the paper would have been a waste of his time and the examiners'. Of course, in a sense (well, one could argue entirely) he is absolutely correct. The maths exam did *not* reflect his mathematical ability; instead, it showed that he did not demonstrate an aptitude for understanding the purpose behind showing the working out (incidentally, his argument was that if he got the answer incorrect then, in his opinion, he didn't deserve any marks at all – again, very autistically logical). If he had been 'allowed' to show purely how good he was at maths, then he would not have had a problem. So does the problem lie with the autistic child or with the way in which the child is assessed?

Concept to question: conforming to a PNT norm is healthy for a person who, by definition, is neurologically different

In a similar vein to the theme running throughout this chapter, the assumption that doing something – anything, in fact – in the same way as the majority is one which needs careful consideration, if not challenge. Being autistic, by definition, means that one is not part of the demographic norm. This is not a judgement, not a value-laden observation, nor is it a negative statement – it is, simply, accurate. Being autistic within broader society is (for the time being, at least!) to be in a minority group. This means that anything which determines the 'best way' for the majority should be first analysed for efficacy and appropriateness before being applied to your autistic child. This includes everything from how to understand (and react to) behaviour to how much sleep a child needs. Of course, there may be all sorts of things that are pertinent to the autistic child just as much as the PNT, but making the assumption that this will always be the case is not a good idea.

Concept to question: just because a person can do something, he should do it

Very often we are encouraged to identify what a child is not so good at doing and focus attention on making the child better at doing it. This is fine – admirable, even, in some ways. However, we must also be aware of what the actual goal is, and whether or not the effort is actually worth the end result. As noted earlier, there isn't anything that an autistic child theoretically cannot do just because he is autistic – aside from not being autistic. But does this mean he should be encouraged to achieve goals that are possibly somewhat arbitrary and, in fact, of little use to him? One example that absolutely stands out for me here is the autistic child who is 'encouraged' to attend assembly at school.

Conversations between educational colleagues

He's at it again. I took him along to assembly and he kicked off so bad I had to take him out. He stood in the playground until he calmed down – funny how he knows how to behave when he's on his own! Anyway, I'm bringing it up at the next meeting. He can't keep behaving like this, he needs to learn. All the other kids go to assembly and don't cause any fuss at all.

At the meeting.

OK, so we need a behaviour plan to make sure that he doesn't disrupt assembly. Suggestions so far include asking him to sit on his hands, letting him wear ear defenders and letting him take a tablet screen to look at. He'll be escorted by his assistant, so if he makes a fuss, she can redirect his focus on to the screen.

At assembly.

He sits, ear defenders on, assistant glued to his side, much to his distaste, and every time his eyes move away, she asks him to look back at the screen. She is holding it as his hands are busy being sat on.

At the next meeting.

I am delighted to report that the plan worked a treat – now he's proved that he can attend, he should be encouraged to do so every day!

The reality: an autistic child having to be humiliated every time he goes to assembly, traumatized by the sensory overload, who can't hear a word that is being spoken anyway and who suffers hours of retrospective anxiety as a result of the stress. Result? A child who is (sort of) conforming to the norm, with absolutely no positive outcome for him – with negative repercussions, in fact – but with an education system that has deemed the situation a success.

Thought for the day: how many assemblies do you remember attending that actually had a long-term positive impact on your well-being?

The golden notion

The point: the child in question managed to access assembly, but just because he demonstrated that he *could* does not for one moment mean that he *should*. It's all about energy – how much energy one needs to put into something compared to how much positive impact it creates. This is something that can be applied across all things autism-related – in fact, it makes up the trio of golden rules! We have the golden equation, the golden concept – and, finally, here we have the golden notion:

**the amount of energy put into effecting change
needs to warrant the intended outcome**

The three golden rules:
1 autism + environment = outcome
2 PNT-based concepts need to be translated before they are applied to the autistic child
3 the amount of energy put into effecting change needs to warrant the intended outcome

Running throughout all of these – presumably obviously – is the need for happiness. I think sometimes that this isn't always at the forefront of all support strategies, in terms of both 'Will this allow the child to be happy while we are doing it?' and 'Will this lead to a happier child in the longer term?' Both are, of course, extremely important!

Concept to question: teamwork or group work is essential and works for all

The notion that teamwork and working in groups is a useful part of life seems to be generally accepted, and I can absolutely understand that for many it is, in fact, of benefit. But just because for the majority it is a valid aspect of life, it does not necessarily apply to everyone. I genuinely believe that one needs to work out what battles to fight for your child. It may be recognizing (taking the third golden rule into account) that while a child *could* be supported to work in a group this might not actually be of benefit, short or long term, for the child. Put yourself into this child's shoes.

I've been on several weeks of 'training'. All about how to put up with other people. None of it actually alleviates any of the stress, nor does any of it actually mean I'm any happier. It's all about 'coping' – why I should have to cope with this agonizing process, I have no idea. I get nothing out of it. I keep getting told, 'Having this skill will really benefit you for future jobs'. Well, I can tell you, the minute I can exercise any control over my own life I shall be spending all my energy in working out how to engage in meaningful activity that actively precludes group work. There are, after all, tons of jobs that are perfectly well accepted where people work on their own, or only have to interact minimally – I honestly don't see why I have to be forced in enduring all this group stuff. It is just not for me! OK, so I can now 'cope'. What that really means is that I've given up trying to get people to understand that it's not for me and that I have just 'gone along with it'. The problem is, they seem to think it's somehow easier for me than it was five weeks ago – it's not! It's just as bad as it ever was. 'Coping' is not the same as it being easier, which seems to be an alien concept to those around me! Of course, now I've gone and 'done' group work – and had to suffer the consequences – they now think I should be well prepared for doing it for life. All in all, not the best few weeks of my life. And what do I get out of it? More stress.

Of course, I am not for one moment suggesting that group activities or the skills of teamwork should be something that is denied the autistic child – for some it may be eminently sensible. What I am suggesting is that for *some* children the effort is not worth the outcome. It is not a terrible thing to want to work on one's own – many people are far more productive in doing so.

It is worth pointing out, here, that the skills used in teamwork and groups are not synonymous to interaction skills; people interact in all sorts of different ways. Identifying that group activity is not something that would benefit an autistic child does not mean that one should ever forget about how to support useful interaction. That way, in the longer term, a person may be in the delightful situation whereby she can work on her own for much of the time and then interact with a wider audience to share that work as and when necessary.

Emotions and autism

Alexithymia – difficulty in recognizing emotions in self and others – is more common within autistic children than in the PNT population. Even those kids who might not warrant a label of alexithymia might find it problematic to understand emotions – which, after all, are extremely abstract in nature. Abstract concepts such as 'difference' have been mentioned already, but it is just as important for children to be able to communicate at an emotional level if they are going to be supported to be happy – after all, if you don't know what emotional state your child is in, how will you know whether the environment needs to change?

Because emotions are so abstract it might be useful to make them somehow more tangible to make life easier for your child. And the sooner you can start doing this, the better! Making emotions part of everyday life is probably a very good thing, but you may need some groundwork first. Questions such as 'How are you feeling?' may lead to perplexity or stress. If a child genuinely cannot answer then this is a question that could exacerbate stress rather than lead to a useful conversation – which is, presumably, not the intention! On the other hand, should a child be able to answer effectively, then that sharing of an emotional state could be extremely valuable information for both parties.

One of the major issues when it comes to emotional labelling is whether or not there is a shared understanding, even when an emotion appears to have a valid 'name'. If, for example, you ask a child if she is 'OK' and she replies, 'Yes', this is only meaningful if (1) the answer is a valid one rather than a response to avoid further questioning (in which case the 'yes' cannot be taken as an applicable answer), (2) the child understands the meaning behind the question (is it OK in general, now, for the past week, OK with wearing this jumper, OK with answering your question, OK with what we are watching on TV . . .?) and (3) whether her version of 'OK' is actually the same as yours. If any of these three are not given the required attention then misinformation may be delivered, and you may end up making the decision that your child is OK when she is not (or vice versa). Either way, accurate emotional understanding is missed, which can create huge problems.

So, how to make the abstract more tangible? This is where one might need to be imaginative! Some things that have definitely worked include:

- number charts
- colour charts
- music
- books
- TV, film, gaming, photos, videos
- art.

These are examples only – and some will obviously depend on other factors, such as the age, development, intellectual ability of your child – but hopefully you'll get the general idea!

Number charts

Having a numerical scale can really help to label emotions effectively. For example, the scale in Figure 1 could be all you ever need to display a full emotional range.

Figure 1 A numerical scale

A range of -10 through to +10 with 0 as 'neutral' can be an effective way of identifying how someone is feeling. Proactively teaching a child that he may be feeling neither positive nor negative – which is essentially an ambivalent state – is a brilliant way of then developing a notion of 'better than that' and 'worse than that'. Teaching about an ambivalent state might be chatting about non-dreaming sleep, for example – again, making the intangible tangible! Then one can explore real-life examples, with plus numbers being positive experiences and minus numbers being negative. You could even make it into an imaginary game: for instance, what would +10 ever actually look like? Once you have done this you can start to label the numbers *together*. A discussion over what you could label as +10 is a fantastic way of sharing meaningful communication – if, for example, you identify it as 'ecstatic' then whenever that term is subsequently used you both know exactly what it means. 'Near ecstatic' could then be 'sublime' – or whatever you choose. The point is, once those emotions have been given a scaled label, you can refer to the chart to remind yourself what they mean in relation to one another, and your child can then provide beneficial and accurate information as to how he is feeling.

Colour charts

This is a very similar concept to the above, but for children who are less keen on numbers and keener on colour. It doesn't have to be in colour – a gradient from black to white, such as the one in Figure 2, can be just as effective as the number scale for children who might prefer this scale.

Figure 2 A gradient chart

The principle is the same as the number scale, with black being one end of the emotional scale and white the other.

Music

Again the same principle applies, but here one could use a piano (or set of piano keys) with low notes to depict one end of the scale (excuse the pun) and high notes to identify the other. This doesn't have to be specific to a piano; any instrument could be beneficial – indeed, music itself could be a huge area to explore in its own right. It might be that certain types of music could be associated with specific emotions; it might even be that a particular track could be associated with a particular emotion for the child – this is common among the PNT and could be useful within the autistic population too.

Books

Books can be used to allow for joint discussion over emotional states. Often in books (or plays, film scripts and the like) emotions are specifically identified, so this might be an opportunity to discuss why a person might feel a certain way, what that feeling actually is and whether the autistic child associates with it in any way.

Incidentally, one of the most amazing sets of books that could help in this area are the Little Miss and Mr Men books – after all, many of the characters are actually named after emotional states!

TV, film, gaming, photos, videos

As with the previous section, this is an example of how to divert attention away from the child. Sometimes discussing emotions relating to self is too invasive for a child, at least to start off with, but identifying emotions in others may be a more neutral, stress-free way of labelling emotional states without having to 'look internally' – so freezing a frame in a film and identifying what emotion a person is feeling, why and how it might apply to others could be really useful. Gaming could be even better, as the characters in games – as they are not real – might allow a step away from reality and so may make the process less stressful for kids who do not like the focus to be on themselves.

Videos of 'real' people – people that the child knows – can also be hugely beneficial. To be able to reflect on a video and actually discuss it with the person in that clip is an insight that could be invaluable!

Art

Art as an expression can be highly emotive, providing an opportunity for a child to artistically identify how he or she is feeling (and this could be drawing, music, modelling – anything that suits the child) and might be much less problematic for him or her than initially labelling an emotional state.

The most important aspect of this whole process, however you get there, is for there ultimately to be a shared understanding of emotional expression. Many might take this for granted, but for your child this could be one of the most important processes you can go through, with very real long-term benefits.

As an aside, but very much related, the development of abstract concepts and an understanding of the child using language is something that can be 'taught' from an early age. The key is deciding which concepts should be taught, as these will differ from one child to the next. Bereavement is one example; death is a pretty abstract concept, and in fact is not something that should be 'taught' when it's too late! Waiting until a favourite pet dies and then subsequently discussing what death means – when the child is at a high emotional state anyway – is probably not a good idea. Teaching 'death' – or 'loss' – without the child really knowing that is what you are doing, so it becomes almost a subconscious development, can reduce possible issues later on in life. One can do this in all sorts of ways. Food, for example, once eaten is 'gone for ever'; one can have memories of it (good or bad), photos of it, even other food that is similar, but nothing can ever replace the exact same meal. Introducing these kinds of terms (like 'gone for ever') can be a good way of gently introducing the concept of death in a manner that is not overwhelming but subsequently makes sense. Incidentally, while not everyone's idea of fun, flushing the toilet is another way of identifying 'gone for ever'!

'Allow' time spent in doing autistic fun things – don't judge!

Just because you may not share the joy that a child gets out of 'autistic fun' doesn't mean it's any less enjoyable for the child.

You may never share a fascination with the way in which sunlight bounces off different surfaces, or enjoy watching the same cartoon a hundred times in a row, or relish listening to the same nine-second clip of music over and over again, but surely the fact that your child yearns to do so and gets so much satisfaction out of doing so suggests that he or she should not be judged. Of course, there may be other – less fun – reasons why a child is doing these things; *but* if the reason behind the behaviour is pleasure then the child should be respected for that, even if others don't share that particular joy.

Others will judge. Many will say you shouldn't 'allow' a child to spend an hour doing the same thing over and over again. They will say that it serves no purpose (or similar). But behaviour always has a purpose. *Always*. The reasons behind a behaviour may not, however, be shared across a wider population, in which case a very different perspective might arise as to how one reacts to it. However, *if* a behaviour stems from pure pleasure – however odd it might seem to others – surely the child should be encouraged to engage in it within appropriate boundaries. I am so mindful that autistic children tell us (often without words) just how much they *love* engaging in certain behaviours – by the duration and frequency in which they do so and in the adverse reactions that they show when we attempt to get them to stop – and yet we often seem not to really 'listen'!

7

Random conversations

Eye contact

Dad: I watch you, beloved daughter, and I watch, and watch. I chat to you, I play, I do what I can to engage with you – and yet you never look me in the eye. I've always been taught that children need to make eye contact, that you will miss out on all sorts of information unless you utilize eye contact properly. I don't know what to do. Why won't you look at me? What should I do?

Child: Dad, stop with your stressing. It's no big deal! Others make a big deal out of this weird 'eye contact' stuff, but to me as an autistic, I simply don't like it and don't get anything out of it aside from a deep sense of discomfort. Mind you, some of my autie mates even find it painful – so, whatever you do, don't try to force me (or us) to have eye contact with you. It's a PNT thing, not an autistic thing. I've also heard that you lot get loads out of doing it – it's simply not the case for us, so there is literally no point in trying to encourage it. Do, by all means, teach me to do something that I can easily tolerate but meets your need to feel like I'm looking at you. For example, I don't mind looking at your mouth or nose or even your forehead . . . but the eyes thing – no thank you!

Why are you ignoring me?

Dad: Come on, daughter, I know you can hear me: why do you so often simply ignore what I'm saying to you?

Child: Er . . . are you sure I can process what you're saying? Coz my reality is that, if I'm super-engrossed in something, whatever it might be, I literally switch off from the rest of the world. It's not a deliberate thing – it's like a kind of trance and nothing else gets through. It's actually pretty lush. I honestly am not ignoring you – as if I'd be that rude – and I understand that it might seem I am, but in reality I am simply not hearing you. If it's really important, you might want to try and get my attention another way. Try not to startle me, though – that causes me so much stress. Maybe try slowly coming into my visual range rather than using your voice?

Come on, hurry up!

Dad: Dude, I asked you ages ago – how come you don't answer for ages? Sometimes you answer so long after I've asked you that I've even forgotten I asked you anything!

Child: Really? I had no idea. In my mind I'm answering as soon as I've got an answer – in other words, as soon as I possibly can. My way of understanding your words sometimes takes much longer than you seem to think. Then I have to decide on the most appropriate answer. Then I have to come up with a way of telling you what this is. All of this takes time – sometimes even a day or two. But time is a weird thing, Dad. You think I'm slow in answering your questions, and yet I think you're slow at realizing when a single light bulb on the Christmas tree has blown. I mean, I notice it within seconds – you take days! So don't judge me just because our time frames differ – just accept that I'm doing the best I can, OK?

Changes in behaviour in different settings

Mum: I'm at the end of my tether! You are driving me nuts! I still don't get why you're so 'picture perfect' at school, then when you come home you wreck the place! No one believes me. It's as though you're doing it deliberately to wind me up. If you can behave so brilliantly at school, why can't you just behave for me at home? Don't I matter to you?

Child: Aw, Mum, you matter the most! School is so, so tough. I spend all my time and energy trying to fit in, because I'm literally terrified of being 'under the spotlight' and being seen to be different. I am wrecked so much of the time, I'm on edge, I'm a burning mass of energy trained on just having to fit in like the others. My stress levels are off the scale. It's a yin and yang thing, Mum, it's all about balance. Having to keep a lid on all that stress at school means I need a massive release as soon as I'm in an environment in which I feel safe – in other words, back home with you. It's the only way I can cope with life, Mum – it's not meant to upset you.

Mum: Oh, darling, I had no idea! What can we do to help?

Child: Well, I need to understand better how to recognize what is causing me so much stress at school. School needs to understand that my behaviour there is in no way indicative of my emotional state. Teachers need to let me do things more my own way, make me feel less stressed about behaving in ways that are just slightly different from the other kids – like letting me sit in the same chair, just little things like that. I'm too scared to ask them and I don't think they believe how important these things are to me. I just want to feel at home when I'm at school!

Tying shoelaces

Mum: Would you please just tie your laces, it's driving me mad!

Child: Well, I would – indeed, I am desperately trying to – but I can't focus on them at all and I can't feel them very well either. Because they are the same colour and texture the two laces become jumbled up so badly that it becomes nearly impossible for me to work out how to join them together – they look pretty joined up already to me! Maybe you could allow me to practise first with laces that are of a very different colour and even a different width or texture. That would really help me identify the separate laces, and once my fingers have worked out what to do I can use that skill on the same coloured laces without having to look.

Walking on tiptoe

Dad: This tiptoe walking – I don't see many of your school mates doing it, why do you?

Child: It grounds me. Literally. Sometimes, particularly when

I'm either excited or stressed, I feel less connected to the ground – walking on tiptoes means there is more pressure between my foot and the ground, which makes me feel so much more secure. It's rather lovely.

8

Education

Your child may not be in education just yet. You may not even have thought about it but it will appear at some point on the horizon, and many of you reading this will have encountered it already. This chapter is not all about how to educate your child, but aims to identify some of the educational components that could require some thought and consideration as you and your child go through the educational system. So – just to be clear – this chapter identifies some concepts that might be useful to think about in relation to education; it is not directly about how to educate your child!

What school should I send my child to?

This gets asked so often, usually in the context of 'Should an autistic child go to a mainstream school, a special school, an autism-specific school or an autism resource attached to a mainstream school?' The answer is incredibly simple: match the right school to *your* child. Do not base the decision on any kind of conceptual 'what is right for the autistic child' – there is no right or wrong answer whatsoever. Your child might discover that the biggest disturbance in the world is the noise of the school bell; she might find that the smell of the canteen is such that the school is the worst environment in the universe; he may identify that there is another child with whom he is so close that his comfort stems from that relationship, not the school itself. The list of pros and cons for any child is endless – which is why your child is the one who matters, not autistic children in general.

The choice of school may change over time; what may be a brilliant school one day might become a disaster the following school year (or vice versa). The school may become a haven, based on a simple change to school policy (for instance, your child is 'allowed' to be excused from assembly). A change in the lollipop lady after school could make the difference between a good school and one which becomes problematic. You may note that most (or all) of the above examples probably wouldn't make that much of a difference to the PNT child – but so what? We are not referring to PNT kids, we are focusing on the autistic pupil, for whom the decision making process is likely to be very different.

Some people will argue that going to a mainstream school *must* be the optimum, the goal; I have no idea why. The sheer number of mainstream schools and the diversity of quality among them will surely preclude any possibility of making generic assumptions about them. In fact, the same could be said of any kind of educational provision! Which simply backs up my point about it being somewhat ludicrous to make general, sweeping statements about what kind of school is 'best' for the whole autistic population. Some might argue that the reason behind suggesting that mainstream is the best place is so that the pupil can 'get used' to PNT kids and learn how to live among them; others will say that denying autistic children access to mainstream will, in the long term, do them no good as they won't get used to 'the real world'. I do not agree. My view is that children do not simply 'get used' to the PNT way of doing things just from sheer exposure – in fact, this might even be harmful in some circumstances. Some autistic children might learn how to *cope* with the PNT way – or learn how to hide their own differences in order to appear to 'fit in' – but neither of these are synonymous with actually understanding and getting along within an environment in a stress-free way. In fact, I would argue very strongly that if a child has to 'cope' then something is very wrong in the first place. I am not for one moment suggesting that children (and adults) can never exist within a PNT-dominated environment: what I am arguing is that simply by placing the solitary autistic child within that environment and assuming that she will eventually work it all out for herself is a (very) dangerous assumption to make.

Mainstream environments

To those who believe that the child *needs* to be exposed to the PNT 'mainstream' world in order to prepare for life ahead, I would suggest that they meet up with a few autistic adults who can explain that, as soon as they were able, they deliberately chose a life whereby such an existence was kept to a minimum! It is possible – not always desirable for everyone but certainly beneficial for some – to live life outside the mainstream environment and to be perfectly happy in doing so. And what is this 'real world' anyway? Surely we should be striving to do what is best for the child, not assuming that he will have to develop the same way of doing things as everyone else? I have had these arguments with people who are determined to develop the 'skill' of doing a weekly shop at the supermarket, the rationale being that this is a skill that is necessary for the average adult. But we are not talking about 'average' – we are talking about the autistic individual who, by definition, is not 'average' – so, surely, the 'rules' cannot be said to apply invariably in the same way! Of course, by all means, if supermarket shopping is genuinely a skill that will be of benefit to the child then go for it, but in some cases it is absolutely crystal clear that the cons outweigh the pros.

OK, so I have now spent hour upon hour upon hour having to learn how to tolerate entering the autism hell commonly known as the supermarket. I have been given ear defenders, shades and a visual list to focus on. I stand out and hate being stared at, but apparently that's the only way I can cope with being here. I have learned that, instead of screaming and running out at the sensory assault and emotional trauma of being here, I have to focus on my visual list and count slowly to ten. I can already count to ten so practising over and over again seems odd to me. I still want to run off; all the counting does is force me to do something else while I remain traumatized by the senses and the feeling of despair at having to be here. Apparently, once I have practised enough times, as an adult I will be able to do this 'independently'. Oh, joy. Will I really end up as an adult willingly walking into a supermarket knowing full well what a horrific experience it remains? Will I? Really?

Three years later, as an adult.

Tap. Tap tap tap. Tappity tap. Click. Online shop – done. Time saved – three hours. Sanity levels – normal to good. Smugness at not doing what I was trained to do as a child – off the scale.

OK, I am categorically *not* suggesting that autistic children cannot, or should not, be taught how to engage in all sorts of experiences (in this case supermarket shopping). All I am suggesting is that there are pros and cons to all learning – there must be. At the very least, while one is learning one thing, one is missing out on learning something else! It may well be that, after considerable effort, a child may learn to engage with an activity – but one has to consider whether the effort is always worth the end result. The long-term impact *must* be taken into consideration. Overall, is this something that we really believe will be of benefit to the child, or is it something that actually comes from a feeling we are being influenced by, that 'most people do it this way so therefore my child *needs* to as well'?

In a similar vein – and perhaps a simple example – is the child being taught handwriting at school. The child has difficulty with fine motor coordination due to proprioception issues, to the point that writing takes her twice as long as her PNT classmates, and even then it is barely legible. The attitude of the school is that she needs to practise over and over again in order to improve.

This may seem like a reasonable way forward – after all, writing is extremely important! I do not agree. Well – I agree that *writing* might be important, but I do not agree that *handwriting* is. I'm certainly not writing this book by hand, for a start! Take just a moment to reframe this through the autism lens.

It hurts. The pencil hurts. Either I keep letting it go as my grip isn't strong enough, in which case I make a mess and the words are totally illegible, or I grip so tightly that it hurts. It takes me twice as long as everyone else – oh, and the words are still totally illegible. This is torment. I am physically suffering to achieve a poorer standard of writing compared to everyone else, and it's taking me twice as long. The mental anguish is acute, and my self-confidence, self-worth, self-esteem and general well-being are taking a nose dive. This will carry on and on – and when I take my exams I have no doubt that I will do miserably, despite the fact that I am actually pretty bright. Hold on, who's this new teacher . . .?

Oh my . . . my . . . oh! That teacher told me I was *allowed* not to write with a pencil and has taught me how to touch-type on my own laptop. I am producing perfectly legible narratives at a rate five times quicker than the quickest of the non-autistics in the class (all of whom are envious of me now) and have been told that I will be given access to the laptop during my exams. Get ready, university – here I come!

Autism and equality

In this day and age, is the first of these scenarios really worth it in comparison to the latter? This seems to me to be a very clear example of what the Equality Duty covers, yet many schools seem to ignore it. Very simply, we need to ask the following question.

Is the child in question at a disadvantage as a result of his or her disability?

If a child takes twice as long to write the same sentence as a PNT classmate and subsequently the writing is barely legible – and this is as a direct result of sensory issues arising from being autistic – then the answer must surely be a resounding 'yes'. If so, and a reasonable adjustment might be simply to offer a laptop, then isn't the educational institution acting unlawfully if it doesn't do so?

The whole point is that these examples could be extrapolated far and wide. Each day for the autistic child needs to be understood within the context of what might and might not benefit him – from a person-specific perspective, *not* against a set of educational 'norms' that may not be useful as a set of parameters.

Inclusion

The above section brings me on to inclusion: what is it and how is it applied? As with most things autism-related, it's not simple. What is absolutely the case is that 'inclusion' is not synonymous with 'integration'. The latter has a focus on integrating the autistic child into activities that the PNT are engaged with – but this may not be inclusive in a broader sense. My view of inclusion pertains to levels of acceptance, respect for who one is, support around need *and a rejection of the notion that inclusion can be understood in any way aside from on a day-to-day individual level.* After all, the things that might help a child to feel included in one environment may not be the same in another. Inclusion – or my understanding of it – means being able to answer the following questions in the affirmative.

1 Do I feel understood?
2 Do I feel genuinely accepted for who I am?
3 Am I allowed to complete tasks (school work, job, things parents have asked me to do) in a way that best suits my needs?
4 Am I respected for who I am, as opposed to being rejected for who I am not?
5 Do I feel safe in this environment?
6 Am I allowed to express myself in a manner that suits me?
7 Is it acceptable not to conform 'for the sake of conforming' so long as my way of being is not negative to those around me?
8 Would I like this environment to continue to be an option for me?
9 Is my situation constantly being reviewed to ensure that all the above remain positive?

What is a suitable peer group?

So often in education we hear about 'appropriate peers' – but, seriously, what is even one of those groups for your child? I am genuinely mystified at how anyone can make any assumptions about the appropriateness or otherwise of a potential peer group based on minimal factors. For example, I have heard (as an argument against a child accessing a particular educational environment) that it would be unsuitable as there is no peer group – in this case, specifically, the peer group was identified *by age alone.* In other words, the preferred 'peer group' was, simply, a group of (PNT) children who happened to be of a similar age – well, in the same academic year. This seems to me to be far too simplistic a way to identify who might be suitable for the autistic child as a peer – surely there are numerous factors aside from age that make for a good peer? In fact, taking a sensible tack, seeing as autistic children tend to have such spiky profiles, then age is presumably a factor that should be taken less into account than many others as regards suitable folk to hang out with.

Suitability for the child should be based on his or her particular needs, taking into account that individual child's strengths and weaknesses. This could cover all walks of life, not just education; see the section 'Wanting "alternative" friends' on page 96 for more thoughts on what makes a peer for the autistic child.

Concept to question: playtime means having to play

There is an almost unspoken acceptance that 'play' is a good thing. People will say that it aids social interaction, social development, social skills, understanding of other children, communication and so on. However, this *may* not be applicable to the autistic child, who might simply stumble at the first hurdle and so may not be able to access the social world of play in the very first instance. If this is the case, then many professionals would argue that the main aim is to get your child to a point at which he or she is with other kids who are playing, in order to 'allow' your child to learn. This is a great idea *only if your child is someone for whom this will be a positive experience*. This is such a massively important point: children develop at different rates, and if your child literally has no understanding of other children's play activity then forcing her into that sort of situation can be terrifying, with no advantageous results whatsoever. If this is the case, then my view is that 'allowing' the child to disengage and do something else that is a positive experience is far better for her than making her do something that could lead to all sorts of negative feelings and longer-term problems. I am not for one moment suggesting that you 'give up' on play activity – just be very careful indeed in terms of when and how you broach it. The following illustrates this.

I had to go to a party today. All the kids in my year at infant school were invited so Mum thought I'd better go, but it was an absolute nightmare. I had to wear unfamiliar clothes, I spent hours utterly stressed worrying about what I was supposed to do when I got there, I didn't see the point of going (I don't even like the birthday person) and when I got there I was on the verge of meltdown the entire time. The noise, the smells, the proximity to others – none of this helped – but the worst part was the games. We were all expected to join in these weird games but no one told us the rules – or, if they did, no one else seemed to follow them. I was utterly bewildered the entire time and made to feel like the odd one out while everyone else seemed to be laughing at me. I just craved home time. Lesson learned – don't ever bother again.

Of course, this is just one scenario, but you may be surprised at just how common it is for autistic adults to recount similar experiences. People are usually adults for far longer than they are children, so it is incredibly important to try to allow autistic children to have as positive an experience of social occasions as possible, so as not to put them off further down the line.

Being exposed to play does not necessarily mean that a child is somehow going to pick it up and learn it via some kind of osmosis. Plenty of PNT children do learn via exposure, but this cannot be taken for granted for your child. So, any reasoning that goes along the lines of 'the more she's with other kids the more she'll learn how to get on with them' cannot be taken as fact. Imagine a scenario whereby the constant anxiety of being with other kids is literally a barrier to ever working out what to do with them – in such a case the likely outcome will be a very miserable child. Identifying positive social experiences, in manageable chunks, while allowing alternative time to relax in a way that suits the autistic child will benefit the child far more than enforcing anxiety-driven social activities in which the child is overwhelmed and unable to learn.

Playtime at school might be fraught with difficulty. As above, if the child is not ready for such exposure then it should be absolutely acceptable to find an alternative, however 'different' it might be in comparison to the age-related peer group. Playtime at school is there for a number of reasons, including giving children time to relax, socialize and engage in non-academic activities. However, there are some autistic children for whom such a time is categori-cally not relaxing, who find socializing terrifying and who have no interest in the non-academic activities on offer. If such a child is not going to have any positive benefit from being in such a situa-tion – indeed, it may have longer-term negative implications – then surely it would be better to provide that child with an alternative. To be clear: while some autistic children may thrive in a playtime environment, some will find it traumatic – literally. The likelihood is that your child will sit somewhere between these two scenarios, in which case there needs to be careful consideration as to how appropriate or otherwise playtime might be for him or her.

Does age matter?

OK, I am not suggesting that you forget about age altogether, but it is true that people can take exams at times that are not traditional. Adults can take exams that are usually taken by school-age kids. Do not get frightened or bullied into thinking that the world will end for your child if she doesn't take her GCSEs at the same time as everyone else. In the greater scheme of things it may not matter in the slightest!

Age does not matter quite as much as we might be led to believe.

But having a contented child does matter. Happiness and well-being are far more important than having a set of academic qualifications at a certain age; having a child who ends up with qualifications along with a helping of trauma as a result of having to gain them is not a goal anyone should be aiming for.

9

Autistic loveliness

Autism and loveliness are not exclusive – why should they be? And yet I did hear of a comment that went along the lines of 'But how can your children be autistic? They are so lovely!' I mean, what an utterly bizarre statement to make, and so deep-rooted in the general level of lack of understanding of this day and age – it demonstrates just how far we have to go.

However, there are some aspects of autism that do not tend to be covered in the theoretical literature – or even in autism literature as a rule – that are well worth pointing out. Here are just nine of them, in no order in particular, and note that the list is by no means exhaustive!

Sense of humour

I have no idea where the myth came from that autistic folk lack a sense of humour – it's utterly ludicrous. What I would suggest is that, in fact, the humour that can come from the autistic person can be absolutely sublime! I am actually pretty convinced that some autistic people are comics as a direct result of the way in which their brains work. Be it stand-up comedy, writing or another form, I genuinely believe that 'autistic comedy' has long been a part of our society – however well hidden it's been!

The beauty of being young at heart

Many autistic children demonstrate amazing characteristics of maturity, seeming in some ways 'old beyond their years'. The flip side of this, and equally amazing, is the adult who retains a wonderful sense of what joy there is to be found in being young. That retention of 'childish fun' isn't exclusive to the autistic population, of course, but it does seem to be prolific in those adults who are content with themselves and with the world. Perhaps when society supports the autistic population more effectively we will see more and more of this – let's hope so!

Honesty

While some people talk about 'theory of mind' and how a 'poor' theory of mind can lead to being 'too honest' – which to many autistic people will be oxymoronic – others would argue that honesty – as in genuine honesty, not honesty now and again depending on the situation – can be a refreshing and useful element to one's character. I have heard so many people saying, 'Well, if you want a really honest answer, ask [insert name of autistic person].' Surely this is something to be celebrated?

Loyalty

Your autistic child or friend or wife – whoever – might make for the most loyal person you will ever meet. Some autistic people (not all, of course) demonstrate a level of loyalty that can be astounding. This may not just be for a relationship, it can be a cause, a person, an ethic – whatever it is, once a loyal autistic person decides on something to be loyal to, there can be very little that will change their mind!

Fairness

Some autistic folk have a sense of fairness way over and beyond what one might find within the PNT population. Sometimes this fairness might have a focus on one particular area rather than a more general sense, but when an autistic person has a burning desire for things to be fair it can be an awesome thing to behold!

Determination

A determined autistic person should never be underestimated! It's not a good idea to get into a battle of wills with such a person – there will either be no 'winner' or only ever one! The level of determination I have witnessed with some of the fabulous people I have been lucky enough to know blows me away.

Friendships

I don't envy those who have no autistic friends. Autistic people can make extraordinary friends – not, perhaps, conventional but so, so rewarding.

Creativity and imagination

Gone are the days (I hope!) when society thought that autistic folk 'lacked imagination' in relation to the arts. Some of the most imaginative and creative people I have ever known of and/or met have been autistic – and this is without even delving into the world of wondering about famous people from the past who, in another era, may have 'qualified' for an autism identification. Music, writing of all forms, art of all kinds – these are littered with autistic creativity and imagination. Science, mathematics, computing and philosophy all also warrant a mention, to the point where one has to wonder where the world would be without the autistic brain.

Inspiration

I am indulging myself here. I cannot speak for anyone else, but I am inspired, every day, by the autistic people I know, work with, work for, am associated with, chat to, engage with online, read the words of and admire. You folk can be awesome. My life is infinitely better because of you. Thank you.

To the parents who have stayed with me thus far – or to those who have simply skipped to the end – you have amazing children who can achieve amazing things. It might take years before you see the fruits of autism-friendly parenting, and it might take so much energy to fight for the rest of the world to follow you in your child-friendly approaches. But every second will be worth it. I am not a good enough writer to finish this book in my own words, so I am indulging myself by 'borrowing' (and paraphrasing slightly) the words of Alyssa Aleksanian, an outstanding autistic writer, who states (in Luke Beardon and Dean Worton (eds), *Bittersweet on the Autism Spectrum*, 2017, Jessica Kingsley):

> The privilege of being oneself is a gift many take for granted, but for the autistic person, being allowed to be oneself is the greatest and rarest gift of all.

Index

Overcoming Common Problems Series

Selected titles

A full list of titles is available from Sheldon Press
and on our website at
www.sheldonpress.co.uk

Lists of titles in the Mindful Way and Sheldon Short Guides series are also available from Sheldon Press.